The Five Senses

Books available from the same author

By Appointment Only series
Arthritis, Rheumatism and Psoriasis
Asthma and Bronchitis
Cancer and Leukaemia
Heart and Blood Circulatory Problems
Migraine and Epilepsy
The Miracle of Life
Multiple Sclerosis
Neck and Back Problems
Realistic Weight Control
Skin Diseases
Stomach and Bowel Disorders
Stress and Nervous Disorders
Traditional Home and Herbal Remedies
Viruses, Allergies and the Immune System

Nature's Gift series
Air – the Breath of Life
Body Energy
Food
Water – Healer or Poison?

Well Woman series
Menopause
Menstrual and Pre-Menstrual Tension
Pregnancy and Childbirth

The Jan de Vries Healthcare series
How to Live a Healthy Life – A Handbook to Better Health
Questions and Answers on Family Health

Also available from the same author
Life Without Arthritis – The Maori Way
Who's Next?

The
Five Senses

If you lose these senses
you lose your sense of living

Jan de Vries

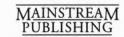
MAINSTREAM
PUBLISHING

EDINBURGH AND LONDON

First published in Great Britain in 1997 by
MAINSTREAM PUBLISHING COMPANY (EDINBURGH) LTD
7 Albany Street
Edinburgh EH1 3UG

ISBN 1 85158 953 8

A catalogue record for this book is available from the British Library

Typeset in Garamond
Printed and bound by WSOY, Finland

Contents

1

Touch

Every time I am in a plane and it touches down I think of the skill of the pilot. Some pilots have the ability to bring the plane to land without any shock but under some circumstances it can be quite traumatic. It has been my privilege, since I was a child, to have flown all over the world. On many occasions I have been grateful to finally touch down at the airport of my destination.

I have also frequently had the privilege of sitting in the cockpit, sometimes of a jumbo jet and, not so long ago, on a short flight from Belfast to Glasgow, I was asked to sit in the jump seat of a 28-seater plane. It was not a particularly nice day and because the plane was flying low I could see the Irish Sea beneath me as we passed through patches of thick fog. I looked at the Captain and First Officer and thought to myself how busy they were kept, during that half-hour journey, keeping that plane in the air. As I was very cramped and could hardly move I did not have a chance to go to sleep in the plane, as I usually do. Instead, I followed every movement of both men. It was an old plane, and it was with great admiration that I observed their skill in landing the plane so that we scarcely knew that we were on the landing strip. Once we had landed I asked the pilot if he was always able to let the plane touch down so softly. He said not always. My second question was how often had he been in danger and what does he do in such circumstances. He answered that you could almost smell or feel when there is something not right. I pondered over these answers at the time and later, when I started to write this book, I thought again about how a pilot must be in harmony with his five senses. If he were not, I am sure there would be real problems. It is amazing that man's five tangible senses are so tuned in to man's technology.

The other day I looked out of a window as I thought about a difficult problem I had with a patient. I thought of the different ways that this patient, who seemed to be a hopeless case, could be helped. To be very honest, all the possibilities that came to mind told me that there seemed to be no answer to this man's problems. Suddenly, a little bird appeared on the big lawn of our Troon clinic. I looked at that little bird and thought of this little creature that had the ability to fly. While it was doing its little circuits above the lawn I thought of that little creature which has the same senses that man has. Suddenly, it disappeared and then I saw the reason why. Although the bird had probably not seen it, there was a cat under the rhododendrons contemplating how it could catch this little creature. Instinctively, the bird had flown away to look for a safer place. Like the pilot who told me of his intuition, this little bird had sensed when danger was imminent.

Sometimes people speak about a sixth sense – intuition – and a great deal has been written about this subject. Mostly it is said that the sixth sense is an intangible sense, but has anything been scientifically proven about intuition or does it just exist in our imagination? It has taken me many years to discover what this particular sixth sense, or intuition, is all about. In the conclusion of this book I would like to explain some of my tangible findings.

When I think of the enormous passenger aircraft in which I have travelled, compared with this little goldfinch, the two extremes teach us a lesson about Nature, technology and science working in harmony together. This harmony can only be achieved if we realise that if we belong to nature we must live with nature and that we are only a minute part in this great universe where so much can be done even with a very small touch.

I remember a patient who was told in hospital by his doctor to go home and live with his illness and I was thinking of the little I felt I could do to help. I pondered a while on the intuition of that little goldfinch and tried to think intuitively and positively about the patient in order to find an answer. The answer eventually came to me when I later saw this man, who had an incurable disease, back at work and grateful for the little I had been able to do for him. He had followed my advice to the letter, and his progress proves that the laws of science are there to help us discover the secrets of Nature and make these available to man.

I often think of people who were almost crippled, living in places where there was barely any medical help and who have gone to a person with little or no medical knowledge who were nevertheless able to help. I have never forgotten the blind practitioner in Sri Lanka who with only one touch of his thumb clicked a disc into place that had been out for years. I saw it with my own eyes. This blind practitioner, with some osteopathic skills, but without formal training in manipulation, clicked the disc into place. Because his thumb was on the right place and on the right energy point, it could be done. It often surprises me how major problems can be cleared by a little touch and it makes me appreciate that Shakespeare could have been writing for today when he wrote: 'There are more things in heaven and earth, Horatio, than are dreamt of in your philosophy.'

Every day in practice I am surprised by what works with a patient, what methods can be used and how little we really know of the human body.

In this chapter I will set out to explain some of these methods. Some of them have been viewed by many as having no medical value, but over the 30-odd years I have been in medical practice I have seen for myself how many of these methods have been effective, and how many have gone on to receive wider recognition. I will say that it is wonderful to see how with a little adjustment so much can be achieved. Life is a constant renewal of cells; illness and disease are a relentless breakdown, and yet it sometimes takes very little to increase the quality of life and improve situations beyond human understanding.

Well over a year ago I was informed that my youngest daughter was pregnant, and her husband showed me a scan of a tiny living creature, no bigger than a cashew nut, at about eight or nine weeks development. Two months later he showed me another scan and I could clearly see a little baby sucking its thumb. That little creature has now become a very big boy, full of life. At the same time my third daughter was expecting a baby. In her case it was more worrying because she had already miscarried three times. After six months it was decided that the baby was in distress and she was delivered prematurely as this was considered best for both mother and baby. When that baby was born it was scarcely bigger than a packet of sugar, weighing all of two pounds and three ounces. But the baby was very much alive. After her first day in an incubator I truly believed that the baby would stay alive. She possessed a tremendous spirit which wanted to stay alive and she fought to get rid of all the little drains, tubes and monitors to which she was attached. This baby would live because I could see that the tangible five senses were in harmony. The breath of life was given to her and that would keep her alive.

She did well until she was about one week old, when trouble started. Her tummy started to swell because her digestive system was not functioning. When the doctor decided to operate I prayed all night and by five o'clock in the morning the answer came to me. Because of my emotional involvement my intuition had let me down and it was not until I had thought and prayed that I remembered what I had written about in my book on body energy: the tremendous power to balance energy we possess in our own hands. I phoned my son-in-law very early that morning and told him to go to the hospital immediately. He should disinfect his hands and then all he needed to do was to place his hands right under his baby's navel. Located at this point is an enormous life centre which not only directs the nervous system, but also has a powerful influence on the digestive system. I asked him to put his left hand under the navel of his little baby and to cover this with his right hand, while breathing deeply in and out. After ten minutes he phoned me from the hospital and told me that a miracle had happened because for the first time the baby had had a normal motion – and she has been right ever since. He told me that he had felt a distinct pain in his left arm and been forced to withdraw his hands. It was then that she had passed a normal bowel action.

Nature will tell us what to do and will also direct us, if we intuitively let Nature work. When I look at that little creature who is so full of life and almost perfectly made, I see once again what can be achieved with a little touch. Her transformation was achieved by transferring energy through the hands, just as I have described in my book *Body Energy*. This energy transfer is neither a mystery nor a secret; it is simply the use of our own power and strength to balance energy. A small manipulation or even one acupuncture needle can balance energy and restore harmony where there is an imbalance. This is often the most important aspect to consider when treating people and there are many ways that we can do it. Let us look further at some of the different therapies.

Just as my son-in-law only touched the little tummy of his daughter by placing his left hand first under her navel and right hand on top, so there are many other simple therapies that we can use. Let us look first at what we can do for ourselves with our own hands, thereby avoiding expensive medical treatment. We can, in fact, apply our hands, so that we can alleviate our health problems in an easy and safe way. Hands have so much to offer – but is our potential for health present in our own hands? Think of how a nurse can give relief by simply placing a hand on the patient's forehead. We know that hands can give comfort and if we look further we can clearly see how much power there is in our hands.

The human hand is trained from infancy to express the thought or purpose of the mind which controls it. The hand is the tool which the mind depends upon when it wants to do anything. Thoughts of action naturally turn to the hand for their expression. The hand is the first means of expression. A baby uses its hands long before it learns to walk. The hand ministers and it carries aid. The hand lifts the fallen and ministers to the sick. It is peculiarly the organ of expression of the good wishes of the kindly disposed. When we are hurt, we instinctively place our hand upon the injured part. When another person suffers and we sympathise, we instinctively use our hand to soothe their pain.

Clasped hands represent the universal pledge of friendship and good will. From the earliest dawn of civilisation, the hand has been used in the most sacred ceremonies. The hand is the natural organ of expression, and its actions are mental symbols to which man has learned to make response through untold ages of experience and adaptation. Even thousands of years ago, the ancient Chinese found that the abdominal area had reflex-pains that refer to certain zones or organs. These zones were charted for posterity. These zones of pain were then known as the alarm signal areas to the viscera which could be developing a state of disease – a sort of warning signal of things to come.

Figure 1 plots these abdominal zones or areas. The abbreviations denote the organ that could be in trouble if a pain develops in any of these areas.

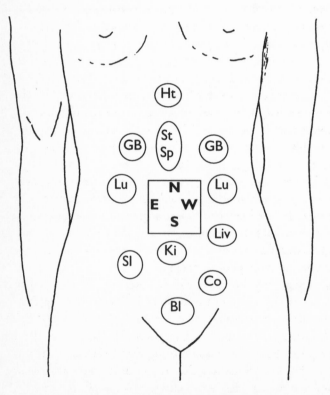

Figure 1: Organ reflexes (abdominal)

Ht	• Heart	GB	• Gall-bladder
St	• Stomach	Sp	• Spleen
Lu	• Lung	Ki	• Kidney
Liv	• Liver	SI	• Small Intestine
Co	• Colon	Bl	• Bladder

To help relieve the area under stress, the left hand is placed on the painful zone and the right hand on the spinal area immediately behind it. No massage is needed – the energy from your hands will relieve and unwind the stress.

FACIAL DIAGNOSIS

Patients often ask me how I reach a diagnosis so quickly. When I worked in China I learned Chinese facial diagnosis, and it is quite remarkable how much one can learn from looking at the face diagnostically. It is possible to teach patients how to help themselves using their hands in different ways, as I have explained. Even a small touch can be of great help. Christ, the great healer, was perfection and knew how to do it because He was divine. He only needed to touch the ill and the lame to effect a cure, and He could even bring the dead back to life. To a lesser degree, man has the ability and strength to help himself and bring relief by using his hands, not only with stress but other physical problems. The reflexologist, aromatherapist and acupuncturist, by using the right points, can often relieve pain, and control long-standing health problems. The ancient Chinese and Egyptian physicians who discovered this thousands of years ago knew that this was not an old wives' tale but a scientific development – and it is one that is becoming more popular today.

Not so long ago I listened to a professor of medicine who knows more about pain than any person I know. He has written books on the subject and during the discussions, which were quite lively, he remained silent until the last moment, when he gave some very helpful advice. He said one thing that I shall never forget, which was that with all the sophisticated scientific methods available to us today, we cannot underestimate the power with which a reflexologist, an aromatherapist or a massage therapist can, with one small touch, sometimes relieve pain where conventional methods have failed.

When we grow old, the white at the bottom of our eyes begins to show. An adult with the white showing is in a very negative condition. His organs are weakened and, having little reflex ability in case of danger, he is prone to accidents. Frequent blinking often signifies the body's attempt to discharge excess negative energy in any way it can. One should not blink one's eyes more than three times a minute. A prominent red colour in the whites of the eyes is a sign of a bad liver. The liver has grown tired due to an over-consumption of food, especially animal food. When the red has spread all over the whites of the eye, this is a clear indication that the organs are malfunctioning.

If the eyes move constantly or are slow to react (to follow your finger) there is a problem with the heart. The pace of the heart is not normal. In such cases, the pupil of the eye will be abnormally large. A moon on the top part of the iris or a white ring around it indicates malfunctioning in the abdominal area.

Swelling around the eyes, particularly a swelling of the upper eyelid, indicates gall-stones. When the stones pass, the swelling subsides immediately. A dark brown colour under the eyes indicates excessive kidney activity and trouble in the female organs. Swelling under the eyes indicates kidney stones. A formation of gall-stones or stagnation of the blood may also be indicated.

Dark blue or violet shadows under the eyes also reveal blood stagnation, probably caused by an over-consumption of fruit, sugar and meat. Bulging eyes indicate thyroid trouble. Pimples on the interior of the eyelid signify excess protein. They usually appear and disappear relatively quickly.

An eyelid that is almost white signifies anaemia. The inside of the eyelid should be red. To examine for this, gently pinch the eyelid and pull it away from the eye. A broad, thick eyebrow is positive; a thin eyebrow is negative. Too much sweet food, especially sugar, makes the eyebrows thinner and eventually causes them to disappear. People with almost no eyebrows are prone to cancer.

An examination of the nose can also tell much about the condition of the person being diagnosed. Reduce your intake of food and you will see your nose grow smaller. Your nose can save your life. A long nose starting high up on the face is negative. A short nose indicates a strong constitution. A small nose pointing upwards is a sign of strong, positive energy. The centre of the nose indicates the condition of the heart. An enlarged nose shows an enlarged heart (caused by excess consumption of food and drink). The nostrils show the condition of the lungs: the larger the nostrils, the better. Small nostrils indicate weak lungs. Well-developed nostrils are a sign of masculinity. A fat nose which is somewhat oily and sometimes shiny indicates over-consumption of animal protein. Red vessels on the tip of the nose are an indication of high blood pressure. Heart disease will follow.

A small mouth is positive. A large mouth is negative. A horizontal line between the mouth and nose shows a malfunctioning of the sexual organs. The lips should be of equal thickness. In general, thick lips indicate a positive constitution and thin lips a negative constitution. The size of the upper lip shows the condition of the liver. If the lip is swollen, the liver is enlarged. The subject eats too much and is prone to mental disorders. The size of the lower lip indicates the condition of the large intestine. When the lower lip is swollen, there is a weakness, a looseness, in the intestines, and thus constipation is experienced. Epilepsy is a possibility when both lips are enlarged. This condition indicates that as a child the patient was given too much food. Lips should usually be pink; however, they grow darker with age. A young person with dark lips has blood stagnation. The blood circulation is poor due to an excessive intake of animal protein and strong negative foods. People with dark lips tend to develop cancer, pineal troubles and diseases of the sexual organs.

The texture of the lips reveals the condition of the stomach. A cyst on the right side of the mouth indicates stomach trouble, acidity or the beginnings of an ulcer on the left side of the stomach. A cyst on the left side of the mouth indicates a problem in the right side of the stomach.

Kidneys: A wide chin denotes strong kidneys. A narrow, pointed chin denotes kidney disease.

Intestines:	Pale cheeks with red spots mean intestinal disorders. Extremely pale cheeks mean intestinal inactivity.
Glands:	Dry thin lips denote under-activity of the glands. Thin pale lips are a sign of frigidity.
Mammary glands:	Lips are usually straight and have no downward curve. Where the lips do curve downward a mother will seldom nurse her babies.
Reproductive system:	Fullness, redness and a moist centre of the upper lip means a strong reproductive system; the reverse means a weak reproductive system.
Brain and nervous system:	A broad, high forehead, fine skin and hair, bright eyes, and the ears positioned well forward all denote a well-developed nervous system and brain.
Spinal column:	The strength of the spine is denoted by the length of upper lip. A short upper lip means a weak spinal column.
Liver:	The longer the septum of nose, the better the liver is developed and able to carry out its work. A short septum denotes the reverse.
Lungs:	Large nostrils mean healthy, strong lungs and also a strong heart and muscular system.
Stomach:	If the bridge of the nose is broad and high, this normally denotes a strong well-functioning stomach.
Muscular system:	Large convex eyes denote a well-developed system.

In China I learned to look, listen and feel in order to reach a diagnosis. The teachings of Confucius strongly reinforce the reference of duty to family and society, and facial expressions and hands, feet or other body readings explain an interaction of yin and yang that produces the five elements: water, fire, metal, earth and wood. Everything in the universe contains these elements. They are not, as is sometimes said, divine forces but forces of Nature and they have to be kept in balance.

- Fire produces earth, but overcomes metal.
- Metal produces water but overpowers wood.
- Water produces wood but overpowers fire.
- Earth produces metal but overpowers water.
- Wood produces fire but overpowers earth.

In the Chinese religious traditions there was a recognised relationship between heaven, earth and humanity. Water, fire, wood, metal and earth are the five Chinese elements – they exist everywhere and are present in everything.

In acupuncture, and also in acupressure, we have to take these principles into account when we treat patients. The different-shaped faces in Chinese facial diagnostics are important in relation to these five elements – and you can actually see the same in animals. Just as the lines in our hands continually change, so do the lines in our face. Even our complexion has a lot to do with this.

MAGNETIC POLARITY OF THE HUMAN BODY

When I see a patient and I look, listen and feel I then ask myself where the energy is disturbed. I feel the five pulses, I study the face, I feel the skin to check the temperature and I look at the entire body to discover where there might possibly be an imbalance – and sometimes a little touch can change it. If we look at the way we should use our hands, this is not only for ourselves but for people that help us, or for therapists or doctors.

Whenever I give seminars on this subject I stress the hand application very strongly. If we think of the battery of a car, it has a plus and a minus, a positive and a negative, and as we know from schooldays a neutral zone right in the middle – the zone where nothing happens. Positive looks for negative, and negative looks for positive. I have told many reflexologists, aromatherapists and acupuncturists how important it is when they use touch for health or when they work with their hands that they use their thumbs, which are very powerful in getting to this neutral zone. Just as the battery of a car can be charged so it is the same with the human body. By placing the thumbs on the right points we can balance energy, even when something is out of place.

I have often worked with copper and zinc magnets, we can also see here that the polarity is important between the South and North Poles. Sometimes I have been surprised at what can be done with magnets as well as what can be done with hands, and later I will mention a few case histories to illustrate this. The workings of the right and left hand can be compared to the battery of a car which has positive and negative aspects. It is the same in the human body when speaking of the different polarities of a magnet.

Bearing this in mind, it must be stated that the poles are not homogenous (alike) but bilateral (different). It has been proved scientifically that the poles of a magnet are different. The South or positive pole gives off a circling form of vortex energy that spins to the right and the North or negative pole gives a movement to the left.

Research has found that human hands also have an inherent North or negative pole power as well as a South or positive pole power. These facts must be understood when using hands to ease pain and discomfort. Please note that the South or positive pole energy is contained in the right hand, and has a tendency to affect a condition of upgrading life, whilst the North or negative pole, contained in the left hand, arrests all forms of life and contracts. The following will put you in the picture.

The use of the right hand or South pole energy: the energy emanating from the right hand will strengthen biological systems and thus produce an increase in general strength. It is worth noting here that any type of infection, bacteria, virus or disease is, in fact, a form of life in itself. *Never* use the right hand on such areas of infection, as doing so would help these infections to grow instead of arresting them. Do, however, use the right hand if you need to strengthen an area, providing no infection or disease exists at that point or area. Remember, the right hand carries a positive charge.

The use of the left hand or North pole energy: the left hand affords relief from pain. It also has the ability to arrest or slow down an infection, alleviate nerve pains, reduce swellings and has also been known to dissolve surface tumours. The left hand is a negative polarity of influence and thus it has the ability to slowly dissolve calcium and any unnatural build-up of tissue. Swollen tendons, weak muscles and similar complaints will show improvement following the application of the left hand to the area.

When treating a friend or relation, you should keep the above reactions in mind. Normally, all areas on the left anterior (front) should be treated with the right hand. For all areas on the left posterior (back) the left hand should be used. The same principle applies to the right of the body: always use the left hand on the right anterior and on the right posterior always use the right hand. This simple logic will become clear if you study the chart depicting flow of energy (Figure 2 on p.21). This method will always put the practitioner into circuit with the patient.

There is, however, an exception to the above rules. When a car battery runs out of energy, the positive pole is connected to the positive pole of electricity and the negative pole to the negative pole of electricity. Thus, the internal body of the battery receives a charge. The human body can be likened to a battery and when it is depleted (has no energy) this same method can be utilised to advantage to start the flow of energy. In these circumstances use the right (positive) hand on the positive side of the body (be it the back or front of the body) and the left (negative) hand on the opposite side of the body (negative side).

Just as the battery is recharged, so will the human energies be charged within the depleted body. In all instances, please follow the explicit hand applications as described; these methods have been tried and tested, and never before explained in print.

Right-hand palm • Positive energy
Left-hand palm • Negative energy

The principle of polarity in the human body is the action of the finer energies in Nature which work like the atomic energy on wireless waves. The radiant waves of this innate energy of life and warmth seep over every living cell as a current which is the prime mover in embryonic cellular life long before the organised 'telephone system' of nerve tracts for specific function and action develops.

This primary motive energy of life is a threefold principle in operation as male (or positive) and female (or negative) and a neutral pole as the child or product, as well as the unknown origin of both poles in the beginning. So, the first is the process of creation in all forms. It is only through the discovery of atomic action that we can be convinced of the actual presence of this function in every particle of matter, including the human body. This warmth of life, like atomic heat, is then stepped down and transmuted into chemical and mechanical action guided by sparks of nerve energy to control its local and specific function.

These finer forces in Nature were recognised as realities by the Ancients. They are the key to the principles of health and their application in the body through manipulative polarisation, the lost art of healing.

The neutral position of the embryo in the mother's womb is the origin and place of building the body by these finer energies in Nature's secret domain prior to chemistry and mechanics. The energy pattern and the geometric designs created here carry on through life and build the nervous system, the circulation, the glands, and the muscular and body structure.

The body of man is a microcosm within a macrocosm and is thus subject to all the physical, chemical and electrical laws that govern the universe. Recent moon probes have shown that the earth has not only an atmosphere but also an ionosphere surrounding it. Different layers, comprising fine electromagnetic energy fields, surround this earth. What happens in the ionosphere finally takes place in our atmosphere. Today, there is growing concern about what is happening to our protective ionosphere. The hydrogen and the atom bomb, and other forms of environmental interference, have ruptured our protective ionosphere; this allows the ultra-violet and cosmic rays to pass through which, over time, will injure the earth's vegetation.

Naturally, you will wonder what this has to do with the electromagnetic field of our bodies. Remember, the human body is an extension of the earth: it has three finer magnetic fields:

- the emotional electric energy field
- the mental electrical magnetic field
- the electrical magnetic field

Actually, the whole universe constitutes a mass of electromagnetic light waves in gravitational movement. In other words, the universe – including the human form – is continually in a state of pulsating electromagnetic light waves as solid and liquid gases, but in reality these waves are continually manifesting motion or vibration.

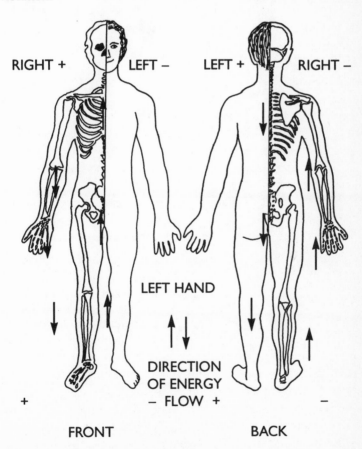

RIGHT +   LEFT –   LEFT +   RIGHT –

LEFT HAND

DIRECTION
OF ENERGY
– FLOW +

+   –

FRONT   BACK

Figure 2: The human body 'magnetic polarity'

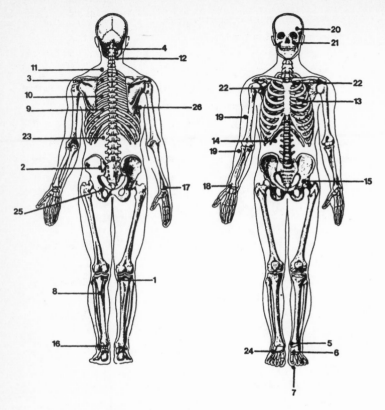

Figure 3: Major contact points

Disease means *dis-ease* or lack of ease or harmony, or a lack of well-being. Emotion means *a moving out of energy*. The body's energy fields have to be normalised or balanced before the disease or symptom can be corrected. Disease is really the result of disorganised electrical forces. Health results in the organisation of electrical forces – we must learn to organise these forces to maintain good health.

The diagram of the human body in Figure 2 shows that the plus, or positive, energy flows *down* the right-side front and the negative energy *up* the back of the right side. In opposition, there is a negative or minus flow *upward* on the left side and positive, or plus, flow *downward* on the left-side back. These flows of body energy are like two separate magnets, giving their respective polarities to the human body.

There also exist some major points of contact which it is important to treat when necessary; believe it or not, there are 22 anterior points of control, 11 on each body. These points are shown in Figure 3 and explained below.

Location of contact area – anterior aspect (*these are bilateral*)
5. On the foot in front and above the middle ankle (between the two tendons).
6. On the dorsal surface of the foot (inside upper corner of the instep).
7. Under the big toe of each foot.
13. In the centre of the nipple.
14. On a line downwards from the nipple at the lower edge of the thorax (upon the last rib).
15. At the crease of the groin about 3 inches from the anterior median line (where the leg joins the groin).
18. On the anterior surface of the forearm on the radial artery, 1 inch above the flexure of the wrist (base of the thumb).
19. At the flexure of the elbow outside the bicep tendon (bend of the elbows on the thumb side).
20. One inch above the eyebrow and outside corner of eye.
21. Under the cheekbone, about 2 inches from the nasal crease.
22. One inch lateral to the nipple and 4 inches above it (between the first rib and the collarbone).

Location of contact areas – posterior aspect (*these are bilateral*)
1. In the popliteal fold on the inner aspect of the knee.
2. On the sacral region 3 inches from the median line, at height of the second sacral forearm (top outer edge of iliac-crest).
3. Upon upper back, about 3 inches from the spine at about the level of the second and third dorsal vertebrae (under the edge of the scapula).
4. On the posterior surface of the neck, about 1 inch from the median line at height of the mastoid (on the base of the skull near the inner side of the mastoid).
8. On the posterior surface of the leg, at about 2 inches below the popliteal crease on the lateral side.

23

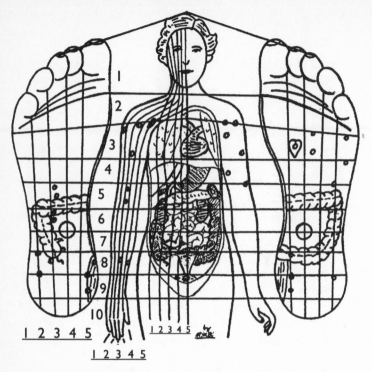

Figure 4: Compression zones of the body, arms and feet
Organs of the body have reflex pressure points in their respective zones
in the arms and feet as illustrated. This is the key note in finding
pressure points for compression massage.

9. On the back, 3 inches from the median line, at the height of seventh
   and eighth dorsal vertebrae (near bottom of inner corner of the
   shoulder blade).
10. On the back, 3 inches from the median line at height of fifth and
    sixth dorsal vertebrae (medial and middle of edge of scapula).
11. At the base of the neck, behind the sterno cleido mastoid muscle.
12. At centre of the neck, below the ear on the muscle near the cervical
    spine.
16. Upon the external surface of the ankle (outer ankle bone).
17. On the posterior surface of the forearm, half an inch above the cubitol
    styloid, between the bone and the tendon.

23. On the back, 3 inches from the median line at height of eleventh and twelfth dorsal vertebrae (base of the rib cage).
24. On the foot about half an inch in front of and below the outer ankle (top of instep on an external edge).
25. On the centre of the buttock – near where one sits down (near the Ischium bone).
26. On the shoulder blade and underarm (go in under the outer edge of shoulder blade).

MASSAGE

All through the ages massage has been of vital importance as a means of relieving stress and tension. Massage is a systematic and scientific manipulation of the soft tissues of the body. Although massage can be applied using electrical equipment such as vibrators, G5 or hydro-therapeutic turbines, the best technique is still to use the hands. There are countless situations which can cause a metabolic imbalance within the soft tissue. Most of these can be treated with massage, the purpose of which is to bring about physiological and mechanical effects. The benefits of massage are relaxation, pain relief, reduction of certain types of oedema (swelling) and an increase in movement. In combination with other therapeutic treatments, massage often provides a form of passive exercise when stretching techniques are used.

In China, massage is mentioned in the *I Ching*, which was written by the Yellow Emperor and dates back to 1000 BC. In 1800 BC in India it was used for respiratory relief according to the books of Ayurveda. The ancient Greek and Roman civilisations practised massage extensively and this is verified in the writings of Socrates and Plato. Hippocrates also practised massage.

Massage stimulates the exterior receptors of the skin and the proprioceptive receptors of the underlying tissues. Relief from pain is brought about through any one or a combination of these effects. The patient as an individual is always viewed as being of primary importance. He is normal in most respects but has developed a problem and so needs help. All kinds of massage techniques can be used; the one used most frequently is effleurage, which is a series of long, gliding, stroking movements using the whole hand. Effleurage is usually used at the start of each treatment to enable the physical therapist to evaluate the condition of the patient. It is then often dispersed between strokes from one area to another, according to the discretion of the massage therapist.

Massage techniques which employ vibration have been developed in Europe and several types of machines can be used for this; massage with certain oils, as is sometimes used in aromatherapy, is also very beneficial to the patient. It is important, however, that the massage therapist has been properly trained to ensure the correct technique is used. There are many different methods, for example the Hoffa method, McMillan's method and Meno method. They all employ different techniques and systems and the therapist must decide which treatment will be best for the patient. The Seriac method involves the most potent form of massage, which is deep friction. I favour this method as Seriac was also an osteopath and his therapeutic methods and compression massage has proved very beneficial for many of my patients.

It was a Dr R.W. Babylon who worked out some of the most wonderful methods of massage which I have been using for many years. One of his techniques – compression massage – has been particularly successful in the past and I have taught this to many patients.

The theory behind compression massage is basically that we have ten fingers and ten toes and we may consider the entire body, or organism, to be divided into ten zones. Figure 4 illustrates what we mean by these ten zones of the body. Each line is drawn through the body to divide parts and organs through which the respective zone extends. The space between the lines indicates the zones as numbered. Locate any of the internal organs of the body on the chart and determine in which zone they are located. Reference to the compression zone charts of the feet will show which part of the feet or hands requires pressure to stimulate or affect these organs.

Compression massage is achieved by firm pressure on the zone in the muscle or tissue between the ball of the finger and thumb. With a slight rotation use a moderate amount of pressure, pressing and releasing over the zone being massaged. The amount of time for pressure on each zone should be from 30 seconds to one minute. The pressure on the zone has a definite effect in bringing about normal physiological functioning in all parts of the body treated, no matter how remote this area may be from the part upon which the treatment is exerted. If you feel worse the day after the treatment, do not be discouraged. Continue with the treatments until all the soreness has been worked out of the zone. In severe cases the treatment should not be given more than once or twice a week.

To massage the foot without using the hands, place a golf ball or other object with a round, hard surface on the floor in front of your chair and slowly work your foot over its surface.

The arches of the feet play an important role in our health. Remember that car you had? It rode smoothly because it was poised on a strong set of springs. We have the equivalent of two sets in each foot. But here is the difference: your car's springs work automatically. The foot springs of your caveman ancestor, as he plodded barefoot through the primeval mud, worked automatically, but yours, after years of shoes and pavements, probably don't.

Now these 'springs' in your feet are your arches. There is the long arch, which runs from the heel to the ball of the foot, and the metatarsal arch, which Nature has kindly laid across the ball of the foot to act as an extra shock absorber. Most of our concern is with the long arch. When we stand still, our weight is evenly distributed over the length of that arch. When we walk, the weight makes contact with the ground at the heel, travels along the arch to the ball, where it is finally pushed off by the toes as the heel of the other foot hits the ground. Or this is what should occur. Too many people fail to use this spring action and clump along with the ball and heel striking at the same time, sending a series of jolts up the spine. Finally, the arch grows weak from lack of exercise and gives up entirely and we have the condition known as a fallen arch.

Ten simple rules for daily footcare are as follows:

1. Scrub the feet with soap and brush every day.
2. Always dry the feet thoroughly. Rub briskly with a Turkish towel and

27

use cleansing tissue between the toes if your towel is thick.

3. Massage the feet occasionally with foot oil, or rubbing alcohol. Very soothing and refreshing.

4. Cut the nails straight and keep them long enough to protect the delicate skin at the end of the toes.

5. Do not do any excavating around the cuticle – no cutting, probing or digging with sharp, hard instruments.

6. Change your socks at least once a day and alternate your shoes.

7. Before long walks or any excessive demands on your feet, protect them with an application of foot oil and two pairs of socks.

8. Give away all uncomfortable shoes.

9. For hot, tired summer feet, try a foot bath made with one cup of Epsom salts and a half cup of Borax in two quarts of hot water. Soak feet until the water is cool.

10. To improve the circulation plunge the feet into hot water – as hot as you can bear – for 90 seconds; then into icy cold water for 30 seconds. Alternate three or four times, ending with the cold water.

Often with massage the power of touch is not only a means of communication, but also an expression of care and affection – this is the reason why massage is of such great value in the prevention of disease. I remember when osteopaths used to be trained in massage before they started to manipulate. There is no better way to release stress, and healing cannot take place unless there is complete relaxation. One of the editors of *Woman's Own* phoned me the other day and asked me what was the most important form of relaxation. I immediately replied that this should be meditation and relaxation as healing cannot take place in a stressed body.

One of the most important senses is touch because it plays a very clear role in the development of a person as a whole. Massage as a very ancient form of healing has been of the greatest help in whatever problem there may have been. Thai massage has been of tremendous help for many people. This form of massage, which has many variations, originated in India and can be used to help and stimulate the internal organs or life force for a strong and flexible body.

We see the same effects with the Tui Na massage, which is a

traditional form of Chinese massage based on the principles of acupuncture. Tui Na helps to balance the body energies; not only does it induce a sense of relaxation, but it is a tremendous help for problems such as migraine, insomnia and a range of nervous conditions.

The Chavutti Thirumal is a massage technique that stimulates the circulation and the immune system. In this case the massage is applied by foot pressure, and often the therapist goes over the spine with the feet. It is necessary to be careful and well trained in this particular massage technique. It works along the energy lines as taught in Ayurvedic medicine. The patient's body is well oiled beforehand and the therapist holds onto an overhead rope for balance.

Rolfing is a technique which has also proved of great value. It was developed by Ida Rolf, and has become increasingly accepted worldwide.

Zero-balancing aims to restore equilibrium in the human body. This method was developed 20 years ago by Dr Fritz Smith, an osteopath, physician and acupuncturist. This is a gentle manipulation method where energy balance is one of the most important aims.

LYMPH DRAINAGE

Another form of massage is lymph massage or lymph drainage, which I learned from Dr Vodder. The principles of this massage are very important and therapeutic, especially with touch or when touch fails, this particular massage is probably one of the most important. We see that the positions are very important when this particular technique is practised. When practised correctly, the lymphatics of the abdomen will stimulate circulation and assimilation, and promote relaxation and elimination.

The patient lies on the back with the knees bent. The therapist stands on the right side of the patient with the ulnar border of the right hand over the sigmoid flexure. Manipulate this part of the abdomen several times then, with the tips of the fingers, manipulate in a circular motion over the descending colon from left to right. Now move the fingers upward until you reach the splenic flexure and, with the left hand over the splenic area (the spleen is found in the mid-auxilliary line in line with the point of the elbow 2.5 inches in from the surface of the body), manipulate gently with the right hand in under the ribs. Then move from the transverse colon to the centre of the body – keeping the right hand on the body, passing around over the head of the patient – and continue along the transverse colon to the hepatic flexure. Finally, continue along the ascending colon until the caecum and appendix are reached.

To drain the lymphatic of the groin, locate the crest of the left ilium, standing on the right side of the left leg with the right leg extended. Press deeply and firmly with the fingers arched in the groin just below the crest of the ilium. Retain your grip and draw the muscles toward the median line counting to ten. Release slowly, again counting to ten. Reverse and repeat. To empty the receptaculum chyli, which is at the lower end of the thoracic duct, press deeply from the groin upward and inward and past the umbilicus.

To empty the liver (three-corner liver squeeze), stand to the left of the patient with the right hand over the liver with the fingers at the head of the ribs. The fingers of the left hand should be pushed up under the costal cartilages. Have the patient empty the lungs, then take a full, deep inspiration. On inspiration, push the left hand up and bring the right hand forward, this will squeeze the liver between the two hands and empty it. On deep inspiration the diaphragm exerts a pressure on the upper lobe of the liver and assists in emptying it. Do this three or four times. The liver is frequently very tender; in these cases the pressure should be very light.

For kidney drainage treatment, or to manipulate the kidneys, press the thumbs gently in over the right kidney, which is generally lower than the left. Then repeat over the left kidney and move the kidneys away from you with the fingers raised. This movement not only breaks up kidney lesions but also abdominal lesions.

To drain the lymphatics of the Hunter's canal bend the right leg with the foot resting on a table; right hand on patella, left hand over the Hunter's canal, fingers well over toward the popliteal space. Push the knee inward and draw the Sartorius muscle outward, working upward toward the groin about 2 inches at a time. Repeat with the other leg.

Stretching the Pubic Arch to drain the lymphatics is seldom used. The patient lies with both legs bent, feet on a table, and opens and closes the legs against resistance.

When draining the cervical lymphatics, stand on the right side of the patient, place the left hand on the forehead and with the right hand reach over the sterno-cleido-mastoid muscle. Draw the muscle up closely under the chin, with pressure on the parotid and submental glands, and turn the head away with the left hand. Continue this movement one vertebra at a time down to the seventh cervical. Place the fingertips immediately under the clavicle on each side and press the thoracic ducts, throwing the accumulated lymph into the jugular vein. Watch the heart action while doing this and do not overload.

To free the pneumogastric nerve, position the patient on his back, place your hand over the chin, pull the head backward and moving from right to left, manipulate deeply and firmly the lower part of the neck on each side of the windpipe. This action frees and stimulates the pneumogastric nerve, which influences the digestive organs.

Draining the scapular regions is done by extending the arms over the head by placing the left hand under the right scapula, with your right hand grasping the patient's wrist on the inside, and giving a gentle traction upward and inward toward the median line. Reverse the position by placing the right hand under the left scapula, with your left hand grasping the wrist on the inside. Extend the arm straight over the head, making traction upward and inward toward the median line.

Stretch the abdominal muscles from hip to shoulder by standing on the right side of the patient and with the left hand on the left shoulder and the right hand on the anterior crest of the right ilium. Stretch the muscles transversely working down over the Sartorius muscle.

For drainage of the rectal muscles manipulate all the muscles over the sacrum and coccyx, stretching the sphincter muscles of the anus upward and outward away from the median line, give a gentle rotation and keep this up for at least two minutes or longer if the patient does not complain. Reverse and take the opposite side.

To open up the superior articulations for spinal drainage, place the right hand on the spinous processes of the first dorsal, opening up the superior articulations by pressing the anterior and inferior with a gentle pressure on the sacrum. Work downward one vertebra at a time until the third or fourth lumbar is reached. Reverse the position of the hands by placing the left hand on the sacrum and the right hand on the third lumbar. Open up the inferior articulations by pressing the anterior and superior, maintaining pressure on the median line. Many operators use pressure to the right or left of the median line and this is incorrect.

To open up articulation transversely for intercostal draining stand to the left side of the patient, place the right hand on the posterior spine of the right ilium and the left hand over the acromion process and make a traction transversely, opening up the intercostals on the left side, moving the left hand downward over the left intercostals. Reverse the position of the hands by placing the right hand over the left ilium and the left hand over the right acromion process. The left hand opens up the intercostals transversely on the right side moving the hands downward over the right intercostals.

To open up the inferior articulations for spinal drainage, the hands need to be placed over the trapezius muscle and scapula. With the fingers toward the seventh cervical, push the muscles toward the median line, superior, until all the slack is taken out and then make a slight thrust. Move down one rib at a time until you reach the tenth thoracic pair of ribs.

To flush the spinal column, raise the patient's body from the table, press the hand on the occiput and bend the patient's body forward until the head comes to the knees. Raise the legs up straight until the whole sacral and dorsal regions are above the table.

For sacroiliac drainage the patient should bend both legs onto the abdomen. Press them down carefully without hurting the patient, move them to the right and press down, then move to the left and press down. Repeat eight to ten times.

To release intervertebral constriction to aid drainage close the fingers in the palm of the hand, thumbs projecting outward. Place the left thumb over the left transverse process of the first dorsal, thumb pointing downward, and with the thumb of the right hand on the second dorsal, right transverse, pointing upward, hold the left thumb and move the muscles upward with the right thumb in toward the median line. Move down one vertebra at a time, always holding the wrist, and press upward with the right thumb, pressing the muscles upward and inward toward the median line. Work down until you reach the coccyx, keeping your movements slow. Reverse the fingers and take the other side by placing the left hand on the right transverse process and the right hand on the left transverse process, holding the left thumb and massaging the muscles upward and inward with the right thumb.

For drainage and to raise the scapula, stand on the left side of the patient, place the patient's hand on the back, palm up, grip the acromion process with the left hand and with the right hand manipulate under the scapula to break up any lesions. Reverse and take the other side.

When sedating spinal nerves in a prone position, if the table is without an opening for the patient's nose turn the head away from the operator, who should stand on the side to be treated. Locate the third dorsal vertebra then place all the fingers of each hand half an inch apart and hold with the fat part of the fingers in the gutter over the laminae with the ends of the fingers touching the lateral portion of the spinous processes. Maintain a slow, steady and firm pressure as you count to ten, then release the pressure slowly counting to five. Do this on all the spine except the heart and sacral segments. Inhibition of these segments produces an opposite effect. After going down one side of the spine, cross to the other side and repeat.

Caution: Never remove the hands or apply quickly or hastily as the treatment will be without result.

Lymphatic drainage should be done by a qualified massage therapist, osteopath or chiropractor. The subject introduces a new approach to some of the problems of structural adjustment in the physiological performance of the body tissues. The skeleton of the extremities is a series of bones and their articulations, limited to movements determined by the anatomical structure of the articulating surfaces.

A striated muscle attached to two or more bones by its tendonous extremities, origin and insertion, by contraction, moves the less fixed part over a range than it moves the more fixed bone or parts. To possess a clear concept of the values striated muscle contraction, one must assume that the muscle contracts toward a midpoint in the muscle and obviously away from its origin and insertion.

Locomotion is only one of the many ways man adapts himself to his environment through the medium of skeletal muscle contraction. The contraction of the skeletal muscles and their resultant movements explain the basic factors in every reaction to intrinsic and extrinsic influences whether smile, speech, pupillary contraction and dilation, gastrointestinal peristalsis or the tiny waves that move the lymph movements in respiration, voiding and natality to mention a few.

Motion through muscular action is the one outstanding expression of energy responsible for continuous activation. This implies a normal circulation of blood, fluids and removal of waste.

The heart, the muscle-in-chief of major functions of the body, moves the blood to the cell. Pressure to overcome many normal obstructions is required. This responsibility belongs to the heart, but the responsibility of the muscles is to return the blood in the veins to the heart. The 'respiratory pump' activated by the respiratory muscles aids in the venous flow from the lungs to the heart. The diaphragm contraction overcomes the resistance of the uphill flow in the valveless veins of the abdomen to raise the blood to the thoracic level and to the heart.

Each muscle involved in the restricted movements of a single vertebra becomes weakened through lack of motion, essential to its own blood supply. Tone diminishes and until the muscle is reconditioned to normal tone and contraction the freedom of fluid flow is obstructed. The source of energy for contraction is nutrition, that is, food, water, minerals, vitamins and oxygen. The absence of sufficient amino acids results in atony or weakness and may lead to atrophy and a sequel of weakness in standing, walking and lifting, diminished respiration, heart action slowing of the return of venous blood to the heart, a stasis of tissue fluids and low metabolic rate. The retention of waste, urea, carbon dioxide, creatinine, uric acid ensues with a gradual increase of fatigue.

Dr Still stated: 'My philosophy of manipulation is based on an absolute knowledge of each and every bone in the body, their several parts in articulation, and their normal movements.' We realise fully that the motion to restore is the one outstanding force-motion that maintains normalcy in all movable parts, particularly the fascia and the tissue, and this motion is the result of muscle contraction.

In summary, muscles form 50 per cent of the body weight. Striated muscles are organs of protoplasmic cells elongated to form fibres attached by both ends, origin and insertion, to the bones. Each muscle is covered by a membrane (fascia). A stimulus to the cell in the central nervous system or to its motor neuron originates an impulse resulting in tone waves and work contraction. Muscle has excitability, contracting when stimulated direct, mechanically and otherwise. Muscles require a stimulus to contract and a stimulus to relax. Contracture is the condition when relaxing stimuli fail.

Motion is the first and only evidence of life.

Normal movement of the body fluids implies that no abnormal substance is detained long enough to produce disease.

When perfect harmony is not found in form and function, lack of speed in motion exists.

Movement is the most widespread of all vital activities. There is no life without it. Where there is diminished movement there is disease; where there is no movement there is death.

Normal motion is the most vital expression of structural function. All movements of the body, skeletal and visceral, as well as of blood and tissue fluid are effected through muscle contraction. A resting muscle contracts five to 50 times per second. Active muscle may reach 3,000 contractions per second – tonal waves. The heart muscle contraction moves the blood from the heart to the cells; the skeletal muscles return the venous blood to the heart. Muscle contraction is necessary for its own blood circulation.

The employment of this technique is simple:

1. Resist the levers to which the correcting muscle is attached.
2. The patient contracts the muscle repeatedly, in time with the pulse rate, and then faster to double the pulse rate or even higher, counting one-two, two-two, three-two, up to ten-two. The frequency at the close should be five-two in five seconds, if this is not an acute painful movement.
3. Press the part to be moved, aiding the contracting muscle.
4. Apply counter-pressure on the part articulating with the restricted unit.
5. Employ skeletal contraction to pump the visceral circulation.

The purpose of this method is to increase the speed and strength of blood and tissue fluid flow, in the skeletal, visceral and nerve structures ensuring nutrient substances can be absorbed by each cell, and extrinsic toxins and wastes can be removed from the tissues.

LYMPH STASIS

The lymph circulation is the medium by which nourishment is carried to every cell in the body and is three times the size of the blood circulation. Any chemical or physical influence which interferes with the flow of lymph or causes it to thicken, produces a most profound effect upon the cells of every organ and tissue in the body.

Under normal conditions, the hydrogen-ion concentration of human lymph should be slightly on the alkaline side and can be tested by the application of a small square of Cantharides plaster left on for twenty-four hours, when a blister will be formed. A hypodermic needle (used under strict aseptic conditions) is inserted into the blister and its contents are drawn into the syringe. This liquid is tested immediately, as the lymph soon decomposes when in contact with the atmosphere. Quite a few years ago, the lymph serum made from a blister obtained from an ordinary Cantharides plaster was used as an autogenous remedy and had a wide range of actions when employed hypodermically.

When the lymph varies, either on the acid or alkaline side, the patient will develop conditions known respectively as 'acidosis' or 'alkalosis', either of which can be fatal if allowed to persist.

The most elementary lessons in chemistry in our schools teach that various substances may be held in solutions of given degrees of acidity or alkalinity. When the proportions of the ingredients are perfectly balanced, the solution may be as clear and colourless as water; but let the acidity or alkalinity change even minutely and a turbid fluid will result, with the accumulation of a precipitate at the bottom of the container.

Likewise, the normally clear and colourless lymph of the human body, following a change in its chemical reaction, begins to become cloudy and to deposit salts such as calcium, which should be held in solution in the blood. The affinity for the deposit of calcium in the joints is too well known to bear repetition, so we can see how these deposits interfere with the free and well-lubricated action of these joints by infiltration into the bursae, and how, over a period of time, the deposits gradually increase, thus immobilising the joint like so much liquid cement, producing pain on movement due to friction which, in turn, produces heat and subsequent inflammation.

Blocked lymph channels prevent the normal supply of nutrition to cellular structures, such as muscle, bone, cartilage, tendons, skin, and in fact every other component of the organism. Even the blood becomes affected. Anaemia is a characteristic symptom of arthritis.

Always test the lymph for excess alkalinity, likewise the urine for excess protein, before beginning treatment. The urine can be tested as described below.

Normal healthy urine should be amber in colour. If it is dark, this suggests that too much salt is being ingested either from the salt-shaker or from salty food. A light-coloured urine may represent no more than dilution by an increased water consumption or an increased intake of foods containing potassium such as berries, other fruits, and edible leaves (salads). If the urine is cloudy it is usually alkaline in reaction, and there is too much protein in the diet. To test for this, add a teaspoonful of apple cider vinegar to the urine in the glass. If the cloudiness clears up only partially add a second teaspoonful. If the cloudiness disappears, it indicates an excess of protein and the amount of apple cider vinegar required to clear up the urine indicates roughly the amount of protein intake.

LYMPHATIC THERAPY

Out of the three circulatory systems of the human body, the lymphatic system has been studied the least. It is true that the arterial circulation is the most spectacular in that the red blood of life is forced through the elastic arteries by the heart. The venous blood completes the circuit as far as blood fluid is concerned. When it comes to the cleansing of tissues and collection of the spent blood flow, the lymphatic channels, glands and ducts play a very important part in sustaining the health of the individual.

The pathology of the tissues is more likely to be associated with lymph stasis than either of the two main circulatory systems. The prevention of the spread of infection is chiefly controlled by the lymph channels and nodes. The peculiar properties of selection in abrasions and injured areas must be under lymphatic supervision or systemic poisoning will be the result. The tendency toward stasis in the tissues of the body that are least controlled by vaso-motor distribution throws an extra burden on the lymphatic channels when the kidneys are already bearing the heavy strain from toxic poisoning.

The physician who can readily relieve renal strain through improved lymph flow is the one who secures the best results.

Take, for example, the common symptoms found when the legs swell during the day and return to normal after a night's rest. This is because the venous system is over-taxed and the heart takes on extra burdens. The blood is constantly being forced into these tissues by the heart and they already have too much fluid. It is true that the skin, lungs and intestinal tract are also active, but that does not clarify the tissue oedema. The burden rests upon the lymphatic system as the kidneys are always working to the limit when pathological phases arise or exist. How to secure the drainage of swollen areas by lymphatic activity is the point that is of interest.

First of all, the outline of the lymphatic circulation must be kept clearly in mind. It must be remembered that the heart and arteries are a part of this circulation. In order to have complete circulation, there must be a starting and ending point. This common area of activity is the heart. The blood forced out of the heart contains lymph that it has received through the veins that entered the heart. The lymph was collected by veins at the base of the neck. The important point to consider in lymph drainage must first of all be the terminals. If these two terminals are blocked it is almost useless to expect results when stasis is present until their potency has been restored. Repeated colds, chills, or an over-taxed system may have caused an interference with the final state of lymph flow into the veins.

Bone lesions, interfering with nerve impulses, may have caused lymph flow obstruction in the thoracic duct or right lymphatic duct. Rib lesions of the upper thoracic area will have the same result. The first rib on either side may be another cause of undue pressure or over-tensed muscles that lie in close relation to the lymphatic channels or ducts. Enlarged cervical nodes behind and above the clavicle cause oedema in this area. It is not an uncommon sight to palpate a visible area that has been causing a backwash of lymph in the antrum. Therefore, the first drainage point to be undertaken is the one at the base of the neck.

The second area is in the region of the atlas, in order to secure a general nerve tone for all tissues that lie below that point. The effect of stimulation, through freedom of pressure, will give results down to the tips of the toes.

The third point is one that controls the flow up the thoracic duct and conveys the greatest amount of lymph fluid. Without thoracic activity, the veins and lymph tracts would be severely handicapped. The chest wall must be capable at all times of raising and lowering itself if we are to expect a return of the fluid that was previously the rich blood forced out by the heart's action.

The raising of ribs and correction of costo-vertebral irregularities will assist greatly in restoring a normal chest action. Starting always with an existing pelvic tilt, make corrections upward. This brings us to the keynote of all body corrective techniques. The sacro-iliac area, if damaged, must receive attention first.

The fourth area to consider is that of the splanchnic region. This includes the solar plexus, semilunar nerve tissues and the reflexes that are associated with stimulation of specific nerve centres. The cysterni must be reached as it is the collection area of all lymph channels below and likewise the origin of the thoracic duct that carries the fluid to the terminal point. The receptaculum chyli collects from the majority of the abdominal and pelvic organs, as well as the upward flow from the lower extremities through channels supplied by many valves.

The fifth area is that of the pelvic basin. Here we find the chief blockage in 'dropsy of the legs', as this complaint is commonly referred to by the layman. The point of obstruction to contend with is that of pelvic tissues when the contents of the basin are already blocked. A sluggish colon may result in a packed sigmoid and congested pelvic organs may interfere with lymph drainage of the legs. There is always a tendency for pelvic congestion to enlarge the inguinal glands. This, in turn, will block the upward drainage of the femoral channels. A clearance of pelvic congestion is essential and a restoration to normal of a pelvic tilt will give the best results.

The sixth area that commands attention is that of the popliteal space. All of the important vessels, channels and nerves lie protected in this region behind the knee. Careful work must be done to prevent damage to the delicate tissues. Popliteal tension may be caused by tensed muscles attached to the pelvic area, and a sacro-iliac lesion will alter knee activity. When the swelling in the legs is below the knee, the restoration of lymph drainage in the popliteal space and inguinal area should bring quick relief.

The seventh centre for restoring lymph drainage is at the back of the heel and under the main arch of the foot. It is amazing how lymph control can be improved by releasing the arch of the foot and carefully treating the region under the attachment of the Achilles tendon.

In order to secure the best results in propelling the lymph back to the veins that lead to the heart, these points of control, in the order given above, must be kept in mind. Always remember the activities of the other circulatory systems and explore the possibility of achieving the best results when each of the three circulatory systems are involved.

MAINTAINING A BALANCED BODY CHEMISTRY

Nowadays we have three enemies. They are three Ss: salt, sugar and stress. Can these affect the five senses and what have they to do with touch? We see that stress is a major influence on touch. There are many patients who develop degenerative diseases such as cancer, leukaemia, multiple sclerosis and arthritis because of twentieth-century stress and negative emotions. I probably see more cancer patients who developed their cancer because of stress and emotional traumas such as unhappy marriages, broken romances, work-related tension, unemployment or financial problems, than any other cause. Massage is a wonderful way to relieve that stress. It is possible for mental fatigue to lead to a cancer process. It is said that a cancer cell is like a brain cell when it becomes overloaded it can cause trouble.

Body chemistry is wonderful when it is in balance, but whenever it goes out of balance there are problems. We have to look at all the ways to relieve tension and stress. It is beyond dispute that fatigue invariably leads to distortion and destruction. In such cases the joints become strained, and skeletal relationships are changed – the muscles operating around such joints are stretched.

The alkalinity of the body is lost because of fatigue. Toxins become acid in reaction and the cellular structure loses its potential. By analysing the distortion and applying certain rules, the body can be realigned, the distortion corrected and the destructive changes stopped. Only then will alkalinity be restored and health rebuilt.

One must remember that gravity is a force that governs everything. The study of the human body from this approach is the main theme of my teaching. The four most essential factors influencing the preservation of life are: food, temperature, rest and elimination. All these factors depend on gravity in the last analysis.

Few people, even those whose business is the study of physics, understand gravity well enough to grasp the idea that every other law is dependent on the fundamental law of gravity. The atom that forms a nucleus and the attraction of a nucleus for its electrons, through the various chemical reactions, is made possible by gravity. Whether we call it force or energy, every source of power – electricity, mineral and vegetable – is only a manifestation, or another form, of gravity.

The fact is that 'energy exists in matter in some form or other'. It is this ever-present energy that causes both chemical and physical change. Heat alone is sufficient to produce physical change in matter, by altering the form of the energy, and this transformation is manifested in a change of molecular structure.

Matter, almost without exception, can be changed by the addition or subtraction of heat alone. The three phases of change are: gaseous, liquid and solid. These are the most easily demonstrable states in which matter exists, but each of these three states is again found in either a colloidal or crystalloidal state. A true colloid, with all its very definite properties, may be converted by external agents.

The tissues of the body are largely colloidal, and the human body and its diseases are our present concern. Because of this, it is necessary to understand the action of colloids and the forces that change them into crystalloids. This change manifests itself as disease. All pain and every abnormal condition of the body is the result of this change.

It is of paramount importance to understand something of the principles of colloids and the forces that govern them. The colloids which form our bodies are identical. Colloids and crystalloids are not different kinds of matter but merely matter in, or made to appear in, a particular state of dispersion and subdivision. The first distinguishing difference between a colloid and crystalloid is its molecular size.

The four primary forces of matter known to scientists are as follows:

1. Electronic forces: these are responsible for atoms and exist between the positive protons and negative electrons of the atom. These are strong forces.
2. Atomic forces: these are responsible for the formation of molecules and exist between positive and negative atoms. Crystalloids are formed and controlled by such forces.
3. Molecular forces: these hold molecules together and are responsible for most physiochemical and colloidal phenomena. They are not as strong as those that form the atom or molecules.
4. Molar forces: these hold groups of molecules together and are responsible for ordinary physical and astronomical phenomena.

The smaller the body, the easier the movement and this is true of the entire spectrum. This is due to the force of the molecules manifested in the Brownian Movement. Some of you may wonder what I mean by this Brownian Movement – actually it is an experimental fact which reveals evidence of the existence of molecules that are themselves inaccessible under the microscope. It has been determined that the same state of unrest and perpetual bombardment that exists between molecules of microscopic size also exists in molecules that are not visible even under the ultra-microscope. The same forces exist between atoms and the electrons that go to seek the atom – and the smaller the size, the greater the movement.

This Brownian Movement is constantly occurring in all the tissues of the body, but in various degrees depending on the fluidity and colloidiality of the tissues.

Adhesion is the term used to describe the property of molecules for sticking to each other. This property is very slightly present in crystalloids and, as it increases, colloids are formed. It must always be present in colloids to retain the necessary size of the colloidal molecule.

In molecular masses, the external molecules occupy a position quite different from that of the interior molecules: part of the attractive force of the surface molecule is directed inward and a residual unsatisfied portion is directed outward. In colloids, these residual fields of force are very strong (e.g. gum, glue). The properties of adhesion and absorption are due to the polarity that is present in the colloid. Chemical action is identical to electrical action, for both depend on the same force of attraction and repulsion – colloids and crystalloids contain this force and energy.

All living matter has what we call *life force*. Colloids are extremely sensitive to the action of external agents due to the softness of their gelatinous particles. The life of the cell depends on the creation and maintenance of an electrical potential and the various functions of life are due to variations of that potential. Living cells are self-caring condensers built on the fundamental plan of the atom, the solution – the colloid. Electricity is the thread which binds together form and function.

In the human being we find the most positive cells in the brain and its appendages. These cells form the positive role of the body. The liver is the negative pole of the body because it collects the waste products. Pathological conditions in the cell are caused by fatigue – lowered resistance of the cells which have been under constant stimulation due to accumulated toxins. The cells reach their coagulation point because the body is not able to rest. Fatigue is then a measure of death. Contracted muscle is muscle on the road to death. Fatigue poisons, whose presence is known as acidosis, produce the coagulation of the cell contents. The level of acidosis (fatigue poisons) measures the degree and amount of disease and the approach of exhaustion and death. Thus, the origin of disease is in muscular tissue.

A perfectly balanced body can stand with the feet together, eyes closed, muscles relaxed, with the bones supporting the weight of the body and without being subject to fatigue. Any distortion of the body structure distorts the balance so the bones are no longer in a position to support the weight of the body and the muscles must contract to hold the body upright and then the muscles are subject to fatigue. Applying the hands correctly to certain areas of the body helps to eliminate fatigue and thus restore a balance of the body energies.

Relax the tissues and the load will be taken off the body and mind. The body feels as light as a feather and all work and movement can be achieved without effort. In this restored condition, all the energy that was required to barely exist is freed and turned into productive channels. It is very important that cellular and intercellular tensions are corrected so as to remove all strain – in short, bring all matter back to optimum usefulness by the correction of fatigue.

Remember: 'All healing only takes place in complete relaxation.'

Dr Marvin Shapiro, a psychologist working for the Metropolitan Life Insurance Company, has outlined seven ways to keep tension and stress under control. These are as follows:

1. Take a physical break: exercise, walk or otherwise interrupt your routine for five minutes or so on a regular schedule throughout the workday.
2. Don't cheat on sleep: try not to work at home, but if you must, then stop at least an hour before you go to bed. Develop a hobby to take your mind off the job.
3. Learn to recognise stress: watch for indicators like increased smoking, additional drinking and frequently disturbed sleep.
4. Stay with a problem: don't switch to something else and leave it unsolved. Step back and reflect on it objectively before pursuing a conclusion.
5. Clarify your personal values: recognise when it pays to fight or when it pays to yield.
6. Face up to your tensions: accept the fact you have them and have to reduce them. This will help reduce organic effects.
7. Plan happy times with your family: do things together that make happy memories. Your partner is your best customer and deserves the same consideration. Call home regularly when you are on a trip, particularly in the mornings.

REFLEXOLOGY

The next therapy I would like to discuss is reflexology. Nowadays, reflexologists are much more accepted and valued as providing tangible benefits to health. I was first introduced to reflexology many years ago, long before it became so popular, and I have seen many of its benefits for myself. Some years ago I wrote a book entitled *Body Energy* which seems to be helpful to reflexologists. In another book, *Stories the Feet Can Tell,* Eunice Ingham tells us all about the subject of reflexology. Historically, the feet have a lot to tell us and they can be used to pinpoint the endocrine system, which I have discussed in near enough every other book I have written. The methods of using the feet practised by the Chinese, the Egyptians and other Oriental practitioners are totally different to those written about by Bressler, Reilly, Fitzgerald, Marie Stoffel and many others. Many methods have been used to relieve pain and suffering but none are as valuable as combating the stress factor through the feet. Many stubborn cases have found relief through foot reflex release.

Every part of the body that is in touch with the outside world has a set of reflexes which reflect every part of our body and mind. In daily life our feet communicate with the earth we stand on and our head with the heavens above.

There are numerous books available on foot and hand reflexes, but most of the necessary information is also contained in Book One of *Painless Pain Control* by Len Allan. It will be necessary to study the foot chart (see Figure 5 on page 50) to get a full picture for yourself. It has been my experience that much better results are achieved by first examining the feet; second, adjusting the feet, and third, massaging the feet. Some of the simple adjustments I use are described below.

The cuboids: This is the cornerstone of the Gothic arch of the feet. To adjust, make a paddle contact with the left hand back of the tuberosity of the fifth metatarsal. Place the right hand over the opposite side of the foot with the thumb under the arch. Bring both elbows up and away with a snap.

(In my practice I have found that if I adjust the cuboids, it is not necessary to spend time on the other bones that make up the foot.)

Calluses and hard corns: These are build-ups of dead skin and anybody can trim them painlessly. Simple remedies can be helpful, too. But Dr Alexander Hersh notes that older patients; diabetics; those suffering from arthritis or peripheral vascular disorders; or others who experience difficulty in treating their own corns and calluses should seek professional help.

Soft corns: These arise between the toes, resulting from local bone pressure. They represent a hazard if self-doctored and should be treated professionally.

Pain in ball of foot: This can be caused by any one of several factors such as neuroma, an enlargement of nerve fibres, excessively high arches, hammer toes or an excessively shortened Achilles tendon. Sufferers should seek professional guidance for proper treatment.

Itch, rash or pimples: These are skin problems that should be treated by those in the profession who have dermatological expertise. But as a temporary measure, the use of a skin conditioning supplement like Derma-Time can be very helpful.

Ingrown toenails: These can be caused by poorly fitted shoes and socks, deformed nails or improper pedicure. The proper way to cut the toenails is straight across, leaving the flanges up. If, for some reason, a nail continues to grow into the toe, or the patient, because of age or disability, cannot cut his or her nails properly, he or she should obtain a professional pedicure.

Bunions: This condition results when the big toe drifts in the direction of the other toes, sometimes overlapping the second toe, and the head of the first metatarsal bone becomes enlarged. A painful condition, it can be caused by wearing narrow, pointed shoes, or by hereditary factors. It should never be self-treated. Professional help should always be sought.

Flat feet: While many parents tend to mistake a normal pad of fat in their children's feet for flat-footedness, this condition does exist in certain youngsters and is generally hereditary. In mild cases, those afflicted can get along on well-constructed shoes and/or a plastic arch support. Severe cases require professional care; possibly corrective shoes.

Once you have sorted out all the foot ailments and replaced the slipped cuboid, the feet will be ready for reflex massage. It has been my experience that a wide range of ailments respond to this type of treatment, with sometimes miraculous results. I have found that most heart cases have trouble in the solar plexus area. Even diabetes has a definite reference to the solar plexus.

There is a principle concerning the three main approaches that should be used in life towards any problems. The hips give us the 'going' principle; the shoulders give us the 'doing' principle; the head gives us the 'thinking' principle. The diaphragm controls the thymus and lung area – this defines the quality of life in us. In addition, an old Indian principle is as follows: all body fluids correspond to the *emotional* principle, soft tissue to the *mental* principle and hard tissue to the *spiritual* principle.

The solar plexus is important because this is the centre of the hormonal system. It has a very disturbing effect when it is in a state of tension. Stress always shows in the feet. They can be likened to a telephone switchboard: when the light comes on it shows which line is being called. In fact, it really is not the light but the circuit – the pattern has to be loosened before any response can be felt.

It is necessary to study the arches in the feet: a fallen, longitudinal arch reflects back to the solar plexus and the metatarsal arch reflects the quality of the nervous system. Nail defects, corns and calluses usually indicate a condition of stress. The treatment of these stress areas is easily carried out with the side of the thumb – don't massage but just use an inhibitory movement and hold for a few seconds – this affects the lymphatic system in the area being treated.

The complaints listed below can be helped wonderfully by relieving the relevant stress areas in the human foot. Figure 5 on page 50 sets out the positions of various zones. Figure 6 on page 53 shows the endocrine reflexes.

Arthritis: Work on solar plexus area, kidney and colon. Also the stomach and intestinal zones.

Allergies:	Work on solar plexus area.
Anaemia:	Work on the spleen area. (Pernicious anaemia is slower to respond.) The spleen affects the intestines and can, at times, cause a disturbance in the colon.
Asthma:	Work on the lymphatic zones, the endocrines and work out the ileo-caecal area.
Apoplexy:	Work on the same side as the brain area.
Atlas and axis:	These can be loosened by rotations of both big toes.
Coronary:	Work on the cervical area of the feet.
Epilepsy:	Work on the endocrines, colon and ileo-caecal areas.
Enuresis:	Work on the solar plexus, bladder, kidney and endocrines.
Endocrines:	Treat all of them if any one is tender.
Exhaustion:	Massage the glandular areas, starting with the pineal and pituitary, and work your way down the feet.
Hay fever:	Work on the area around the big toe.
Hypo and Hypertension:	Head zones, could be due to prostate, kidney or solar plexus. Treat accordingly.
Hips:	Treat the shoulder joint on same side, also around onto the ankle.
Knees:	Work on the elbow joints, also the sacral area of the foot.
Lack of energy:	Treat the liver area – proceed gently and cautiously.
Muscle tone:	To increase, treat the suprarenals.
Nerve tension:	Work on the lymphatic area, the solar plexus and the endocrines.
Sinus:	This responds to treatment on the ileo-caecal valve area, also the sinus areas of the feet.
Insomnia:	Work on the suprarenals and solar plexus (effective in cases of extreme tiredness).
Tonsillitis:	Work on lymphatic drainage area and on outer ankle area.

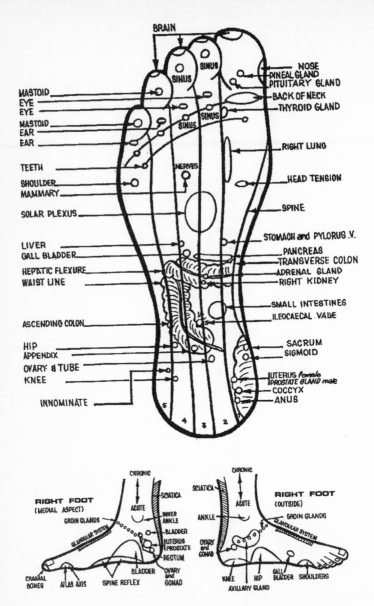

Figure 5: Compression zone reflex chart

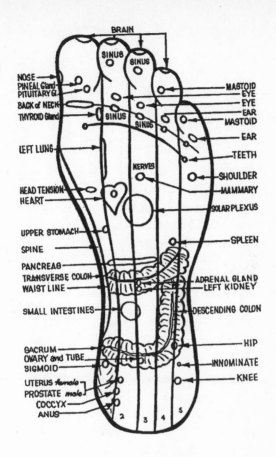

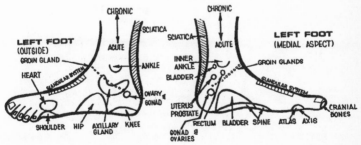

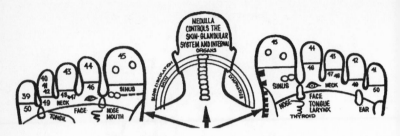

Body zone reflexes

39	Medulla oblongata	
40	Perversion-hallucination	
41	Hysteria-curea	
42	Sexual-life-mentality	
43	Apprehension	
44	Ataxia-motor control	
45	Pineal gland	Fatigue
	Pituitary gland	
46	Visual area	For optic nerve inco-ordination
47	Apoplexy	
48	Speech centre	Epilepsy Fainting Dizzyness
49	Auditory Area	
50	Will ideation	Intellect

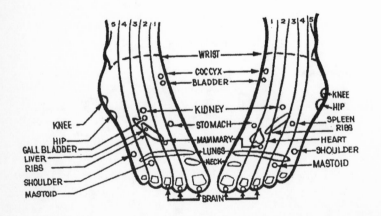

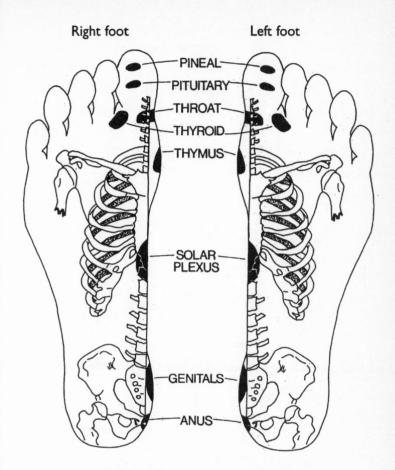

Right foot   Left foot

PINEAL
PITUITARY
THROAT
THYROID
THYMUS

SOLAR
PLEXUS

GENITALS

ANUS

Figure 6: The endocrine reflexes

Varicose veins: Work on the colon area – do not touch the
veins themselves.

It has often been found that kidney and prostate trouble can be the underlying cause of rheumatic pain. In cases of migraine, it would be advisable to look at the pituitary and gall-bladder areas on the feet.

In conclusion, the principle of foot compression should not be confused with the ordinary form of massage. A totally different principle is involved, as the foot should not be stroked but an applied pressure should be employed with the thumb. If the pain increases after giving foot reflex treatment, it is a sign that some pathological symptoms may be involved in the reflexed zones.

The simplicity of these methods should command your attention. Always remember that the more simple the technique, the more effective the results.

BODY ENERGY BALANCE (TOUCH METHOD)

The following points are worth remembering for successful treatment:

To *stimulate* the energies in the body, the method used is similar to charging the human battery. The positive (right) hand is always applied to the positive (right) side, i.e. the right hand on the right side (front of body) and the right hand on the positive left (back of the body). Also the negative (left) hand is applied to the negative left (front) of the body and the negative (left) hand on the negative (back) of the right side of the body (refer to Figure 2 on page ??).

To *sedate* the energies, the contact must be made to continue the flow of energies: the positive (right) hand on the negative (left) front of body or on the negative (back) on the right side. Also the negative (left) hand on the positive front (right side) and on the positive (left side) back of the body.

Never apply too much pressure. *Do not* rub or massage the area – just hold firmly with whole hand, or with the thumb of the hand, as required.

Energy, which is generated by the practitioner, flows into the patient because of the physical contact. So energy flows through the skin, penetrating deep into the tissue, then flowing back to the point of contact.

The duration of treatment for each area can vary from two to five minutes. The total time of each treatment on various areas should not exceed 30 minutes at any one session. The practitioner must not exhaust his own energy.

With these methods of using the hands, you will observe that at times one puts the right hand on the left side and left hand on the right side. In addition to this, when the practitioner is giving a set treatment, he is able to replenish the patient's body energy with his own energy by also placing his right hand on the patient's right hand, and his left hand on the patient's left hand – whichever side the patient is told to apply his hands. In this way, the patient's body energy is enhanced by the practitioner's body energy. This provides a very powerful combination for helping the sick.

There is no doubt that these body energies do exist and do work to heal: every organ, tissue, muscle, bone, etc. has a direct or indirect contact with the surface area of the human body.

There has been a great deal of literature on treatment by using the reflexes of the feet. For many years, I used these foot reflex methods but only seemed to have achieved partial success. It was only when I researched the body zones and the occiput that I achieved a greater degree of success and the patient found greater relief after the first few treatments.

As I have already stated, the head represents the positive pole and the feet the negative pole, while the hands are neutral. It is only when the whole body is balanced that success may be achieved.

A brief history of the feet in healing will enlighten you. Centuries ago, the Chinese and the Indonesians used the feet for diagnosis and treatment. This was their method of exciting the reflexes, of awakening the responses. Even acupuncture is a reflex treatment and acts through the autonomic system. Even if some acupuncturists disagree, this is a fact and a law – the sooner this fact of reflex action is accepted, the sooner their labours will be rewarded.

In my early days I learnt a lot by holding my patient's feet – the corns, the calluses, the hammer toes, the bunions, all these tell a tale. They tell us there are some coherent distortions in the body. Strangely enough, from studying the feet one can even discern the patient's personality and learn their attitudes to life in general. I may even state that inherited factors show in the feet, as every part of the body is in touch with the world around and these experiences are reflected through the body and mind. All matter settles at its lowest point: in this instance, the feet (the negative pole).

As I have already said, in the feet we find all the hormonal reflexes, so I will now spend some time giving some useful information on these glands or chakras, as the feet are one of the most important areas to stimulate or relax the secretions of these hormonal glands.

THE MIRACLE-WORKING SYSTEM OF THE BODY – THE ENDOCRINE AND OTHER GLANDS

The science of endocrinology embraces the internal secretions of all the ductless glands and thus merits our serious attention. The secretions from these glands discharge straight into the bloodstream; they are very potent and essential to the body for its daily use. The ductless glands are the supply depot for the living organism. They regulate the nutrition we obtain from our food. Our entire physical life is regulated by these all-important glands or centres, even to the kind of skin, the colour of hair, the strength of muscles, etc. Many of the glands do have ducts and produce internal and external secretions, e.g. the liver, pancreas, and membranes of the stomach and intestines. These, together with endocrine glands, are listed below. They should be studied further from the point of view of the electrical potential of the human body.

Pineal	Suprarenals or adrenals
Pituitary	Gonads
Parotid gland	Liver
Thyroid	Duodenum
Parathyroid	Prostate (in males)
Thymus	Mammary (in females)
Pancreas	Stomach
Spleen	

The pineal

Drawn an imaginary line over the head from the top of the ears and another imaginary line from the tip of the nose to the occipital protuberance. The place where these imaginary lines cross is as close as you will get to the position of the pineal gland. Very little is known of this gland but it is often mentioned in relation to metaphysics. The pineal gland is known to secrete a fluid which assists in the growth and development of the sexual organs.

The pituitary
This is localised at the nasal suture – the place where the nose meets the forehead. Just behind this junction is a saddle called the *selle turica*. It consists of two lobes:

- the anterior regulates hair growth and fatty conditions. It is also an important factor in the growth of children. If there is an imbalance, this can lead to impotence in the male and irregular periods in women. It can even be the cause of excessive sugar (diabetes).
- the posterior lobes produce a secretion also which acts as a tonic to the blood and stimulates the intestines, promoting good digestion. Its imbalance can cause disturbances in the nervous system and digestive organs; even low blood pressure may result with a degree of drowsiness.

Parotid gland
Situated directly above and a little behind the parathyroid, this gland is important to the sense of hearing.

The thyroid
Situated in front of the trachea, this gland influences the metabolic processes which ultimately affect the whole nervous system. It furnishes energy to the body, without which the digestion and assimilation of food would not take place.

The parathyroid
There are four of these and they are situated in pairs on the surface of each lobe of the thyroid. They produce very potent secretions which help in the distribution of calcium salts which are essential to the body. It regulates the body weight. Almost all glands depend on the parathyroid for their function.

The thymus
This is known as the gland of growth, and is situated in the thorax, a little below the thyroid. It seems to operate until the time of

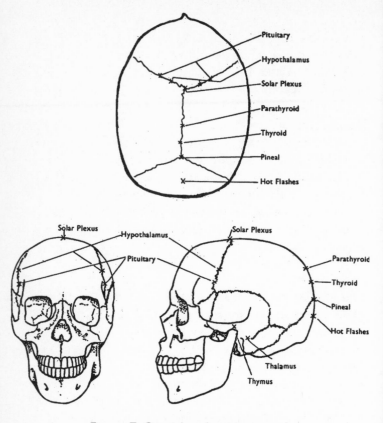

Figure 7: Cranial endocrine zones

puberty. Its main function is the distribution of calcium to the body structure.

The pancreas

This gland resembles a bunch of grapes, and is situated across the posterior wall of the abdomen and has an external secretion known as the pancreatic fluid. It also has an internal secretion through the Islets of Langerhans which helps to change the glucose of the blood into a form that the body tissues are able to use.

The spleen

This is situated directly below the diaphragm. Its main purpose is the regulation of the metabolic process and largely depends on the thyroid for this purpose. The spleen is related to the organs of digestion, assimilation and elimination. In an indirect way, it supplies the necessary stimulant to the stomach and intestinal tract.

The suprarenals or adrenals

The suprarenal or adrenal glands are small, yellowish, triangular-shaped bodies situated one above each kidney. Their functions are similar and related to the autonomic nervous system and their adrenalin secretions regulate the blood pressure. These adrenals provide an element in the blood which helps the process of oxidisation and thus keeps the circulation flowing at the proper pressure. If inadequate, the blood pressure is often low, the nervous system is depressed and death can soon follow.

The gonads

These are the reproductive organs of the body. These comprise two testes in the male, and two ovaries in the female. Their internal secretions are poured into the blood, stimulating and revitalising all the other glands and organs of the body. In co-operation with these gonads, there are epididymis, the ductless vas deferens and the vesicula seminalis; also the ejaculatory duct and the prostate and penis. The cells (seeds) in these glands send out their secretion to the body and thus it is said to be an external secretion.

The liver

This is the largest gland in the body, in both humans and animals. It is the seat of some of the body's most important functions. The liver is reddish-brown in colour and weighs from three to four pounds. It is mainly concerned with the secretion of a thin yellow-ish-brown fluid, of a bitter taste and of a slightly alkaline reaction, called bile. The liver has a very intricate structure; it is composed of a great multitude of blood vessels, nerves and bile ducts and is covered with thin serous membrane. It differs from any of the other organs and has a peculiarity to itself. It receives both arterial and venous blood. The bile ducts originate in minute branches in the interior of the liver, uniting together until they eventually empty into the gall-bladder. This gland is pear-shaped with the larger extremity hanging below the lower edge of the liver.

The duodenum

When our food has been reduced by the saliva and gastric juices to a flour-like substance, it is then discharged into this organ. It eventually reaches the mouth of the gall-bladder and thus stimulates it into action, causing its fibrous coating to contract and pour out the bile into the duodenum. Here the bile mixes with the food and converts its oily or fatty substances into a creamy mass, fit to be absorbed into the blood.

When the glands are starved there is a tendency to stricture, ossification, hardening, arteriosclerosis, rheumatism, etc., as well as consolidation in nerve or brain matter or in spinal bones, resulting in poor hearing, hardening in the strictures of the eyes, arthritis and uratic crystallisation. The results of this starvation or imbalance are often evident in poor elimination, constipation, anaemic blood, feeble-mindedness, etc.

It is worth summarising here how these glands react to stimulation:

Pineal:	Growth and development of sexual organs.
Pituitary:	Posterior lobe – brain, rhythm, skin, frame, gonads.
	Anterior lobe – brain, sex, weight.
Parotid:	Relaxes middle ear, increases secretion.
Thyroid:	The lymphatic system, skin and gonads.
Parathyroid:	Thyroid imbalance, calcium stabiliser.
Thymus:	Controls growth from infancy to puberty.
Pancreas:	Promotes pancreatic.
Spleen:	Regulates the metabolic process.
Suprarenals or adrenals:	Regulates blood pressure, vasomotor control.
Gonads:	Stimulates and revitalises other glands and organs.

Liver:	Promotes bile.
Duodenum:	Promotes digestion.
Mammary:	Develops and promotes secretion.
Stomach:	Discharges gas, promotes secretion.

While I have been writing on this subject I have been looking at the compression zone chart (Figure 5 on page 50) that was so well compiled by my great friend Dr Leonard Allan, who was one of the greatest practitioners of our times. This has led me to reflect with deep gratitude on how he reached a very old age before his sad death just recently. He has left behind a tremendous knowledge that I am sharing with you in this book of methods and therapies. Thanks to his wonderful mind he has left a great inheritance to all medical practitioners. While we can, we have to continue working and using the knowledge he has passed on to us.

The different methods developed by Dr Allan have proved a blessing for many and it was his wish that they be shared. He taught us the zone reflexes and the pressure techniques on the whole surface of feet and hands. When working in those areas he would emphasise the importance of relaxation, improving the blood supply and nerve function, normalising the body functions and never forgetting that the endocrine system is one of the most important systems in the human body.

I have often mentioned in my books that there are seven endocrine glands, seven colours in the rainbow, seven light receptors in the retina of the eye and seven steps in a musical octave. They all have to be in harmony and if one is out of harmony, so is the whole body. We see with reflexology how much can be done with these seven endocrine glands to bring them back into harmony and, further on in the book, when I explore further the endocrine system, we can see how essential it is that these seven small glands in the body need to be in harmony. This is why Eunice Ingham developed the zone theory into foot reflexology. She observed that congestion and tension in any part of the foot mirrors the congestion corresponding to any part of the body. While the body has the ability to heal itself, if there is an imbalance, this vital energy can be released and restored to maintain the body's natural equilibrium.

OSTEOPATHY

Osteopathy, which is probably my main practice, has helped people tremendously to restore their sense of touch. This can sometimes be achieved by relieving the third cervical vertebra. In my book *Neck and Back Problems* I have described the many methods that we use and have given many examples of where and how osteopathy can work. In this system of medicine, which places the emphasis on the relationship between structural integrity and health, where the body is endowed with the means of sustaining optimum health, this can be impaired by mechanical defect. Defects usually come within the category of orthopaedic lesions while the osteopathic lesion may in itself be very minor and difficult to detect.

Frequently, such lesions are nothing more than loss of joint tolerance which may give rise to joint pain and limitation of movement. Although osteopathy is most often used to treat musculo-skeletal problems it is also employed effectively for other disorders and it is well established that manipulation of the spine can alter neuro-endocrine and neuro-visceral activity and does affect general health. Osteopaths traditionally regard the vascular system as being of prime importance and employ a fair amount of soft tissue manipulation. Some methods of touch, for people who have a problem of losing feeling, are helpful. For instance, cranial osteopathy has been of very great help to many people. This is a branch of osteopathy which is luckily becoming better known and more widely accepted.

Cranial osteopathy is really the keynote to all healing. If you can learn the location of the endocrine zones on the human skull (the cranium) and also learn to apply the simple technique of balance, then miracles can happen.

Do not be afraid to use these methods of endocrine (energy) balance, because no harm can be caused by doing so. Unlike the use of drugs or hormone extracts, this method will only excite the glands to function and not over-function. If some of the glands do over-function, this same simple application will restore the glands to their normal function.

With cranial osteopathy, the method of application and use is closely related to the endocrine zones of the human feet. Always remember that one uses the right hand (thumb) on the left foot and the left hand (thumb) on the zones of the cranium. After doing this for a few minutes, change over and apply the opposite hands, i.e. left hand (thumb) to zones on the right foot and right hand (thumb) on the cranial zone.

In this way, pure and simple energy balance can be initiated by the simple application of the human thumbs.

ACUPUNCTURE

This Oriental form of therapy, which has been practised for many centuries, has given countless people tremendous relief. This method is achieved by inserting fine needles into the various active points in the body and is based upon the principle of being a continuous generation and flow of life-force energy throughout the body. This force has two polarities which alternate rhythmically every twenty-four hours, flowing in paths, or meridians, which are traceable on the skin. On each meridian there are acupuncture points which are stimulated by acupuncture needles, thus influencing the appropriate body organs, nervous system, or affected area. The number of treatments required will vary depending upon the nature of the problem. People I have treated for loss of touch in a harmonious acupuncture module have been greatly helped.

The practitioner must decide which points to use. Sometimes I have used homoeopuncture, dipping the needle in certain homoeopathic extracts to help the condition; this too is one of the main principles of the treatment we employ in our clinics. The therapist will choose the points to restore body balance and to restore the five senses to harmony.

HOMOEOPATHY

Homoeopathy is a method based on the principle *like cures like*. It was first formulated by Samuel Hahnemann, and his system has now developed into a complete medical treatment. This principle concurs with what was then the current explanation for the action of allopathic drugs. Hahnemann decided to examine their effect on perfectly healthy people. He tried the drug Cinchona on himself and was amazed to discover that it produced in him the very symptoms of the disease which it was being used to cure. He repeated the experiment using different drugs on other volunteers and his findings led to the reiteration of the great healing principle once pronounced by Paracelsus *'Similia similibus curentur'*. Remedies diluted one part in one hundred more than thirty times over became commonplace in homoeopathic prescribing, which led to ridicule from allopathic doctors and conventional scientists, who claimed that none of the original substances could possibly remain. Homoeopaths were not so ignorant as to be unaware of this, but they understood that the healing force was unlocked when a substance was succussed and diluted.

So often when harmonising the three bodies – mental, physical and emotional – homoeopathy has proved a valuable method for restoring what was out of touch.

VITAMIN, MINERAL AND TRACE ELEMENT THERAPY

In today's society there are an increasing number of allergies and problems of the immune system which affect the senses and this form of treatment is most important for countering deficiencies. In several case histories below I shall discuss what has been introduced and the powerful range of remedies which have been of tremendous help to countless individuals.

PHYTOTHERAPY OR HERBAL MEDICINE

This is really a form of naturopathic treatment and all the medicines are of entirely natural origin. Diagnosis and treatment relate to the individual rather than to a named disease. Allopathic treatment might comprise a single drug for a specific condition, but herbal treatment will work mildly and gently to rebalance the body, ensuring there are no toxic effects. There is energy inside every human body which science is unable to quantify or explain. Herbalists describe it as the vital force which inspires the body to life and is chiefly concerned with maintaining its equilibrium. If this delicate balance is encouraged, then the whole person enjoys good health. If it is disturbed, the result is disease.

Herbalism treats the patient, not the disease, by directing the vital force and encouraging it with herbal remedies which stimulate the body's own defences to produce the desire to return to positive health.

MUSCLE TESTING OR KINESIOLOGY

This method can be used very successfully in testing the muscles for allergic reactions, especially those characterised by loss of grip or touch and specifically in relation to the hands and feet.

CASE HISTORIES

A male patient of about forty years of age presented me with one of the most extreme cases that I had come across in all my years of practice. He started by telling me that he had multiple sclerosis (MS). The diagnosis was not confirmed and he refused a lumbar puncture, but nevertheless there were some white patches on the MRI scan. He did not exhibit any of the classical symptoms of MS. He had been told that he had no choice but to live with it, but his main problem was that he had lost his sense of touch and the grip in his hands. That made his work as a dentist completely impossible.

I felt very sorry for this gentleman, and asked him to tell me the full story. He told me that he knew exactly the place, the day and the time that he lost his grip. He went on to tell me that he was playing the piano in the evening and suddenly a piano string snapped. From that moment he lost his grip. He went from bad to worse and, eventually, after seeing his doctor, saw a neurologist. The neurologist listened to his story, checked him out, and said he suspected he had multiple sclerosis. The tests were not fully conclusive and so finally he came to see me.

I was interested because in the particular area where he lived I knew there was a fault in the earth's surface. I also knew that there had been an earthquake, very minor but nevertheless confirmed in Scottish history and the story of the piano led me to look more closely at the area where he lived. Investigation confirmed his story. I decided to treat him with acupuncture, which helped up to a point; he felt better but did not regain his grip or sense of touch. I then used my intuition and suspected that, as a dentist, he had been working with amalgam, silver and mercury substances for dental fillings, so I decided to detoxify him completely. I used a few very strong detoxifiers. There is a remedy from Nature's Best which is excellent for detoxifying called Multi Guard. Because of its high selenium content it served the purpose. I also used *Gingko biloba*, which is a Bioforce product and most extensively used for blood circulation problems. I also used 2,000 mg of Evening Primrose Oil. It was quite surprising how his touch slowly returned. He is one of my most grateful patients and is now fully back in practice. I have converted him to not putting amalgam fillings into people's teeth; instead he uses composite fillings!

Then there was a 61-year-old lady who was a bit of a mystery. She had a very slight tremor, but luckily she was not diagnosed as having Parkinson's disease. She told me that after an accident she started to feel very insecure with a tendency to start shaking, and this had left her without any sense of touch. She was very annoyed about it and asked me to have a good look at her. I used Chinese facial diagnosis and saw that she was very slightly distorted. After further examination I found that her third cervical vertebra was out of place. Rotation was minimal and I carefully adjusted the vertebra, which gave her almost immediate relief. However, I did not feel that the motor nerves were involved and so I decided to do a few blood tests. This showed that the level of lead in her blood was too high and therefore I put her on a strong detoxifier called CPS. This is an American product, which provides fifteen powerful antioxidants in a base of herbal extracts and other natural compounds. Beta carotene, vitamin E, vitamin C, selenium, zinc and manganese all have antioxidant functions. Procyanidolic oligomers (PCO) from grape seeds and green tea extract are fifty to two hundred times more potent than vitamin E. Concentrated extracts of cabbage, garlic, ginger and klamath blue-green algae are rich dietary sources of antioxidant nutrients. These are just a few of the reasons CPS is the most comprehensive antioxidant formula available.

I prescribed CPS in combination with Calcium/Magnesium Balance from Nature's Best; this is an excellent product, especially when there is a slight tremor. Along with these two remedies I also prescribed Echinaforce from Bioforce to help her immune system. Echinaforce is a unique formula which was formulated by Dr Vogel many years ago. It works very well as a fresh herb preparation for non-specific stimulant therapy. Echinaforce brings about an increase in the body's own resistance in cases of inflammation or infection, susceptibility to colds and other infections. When it is taken internally for the treatment of certain dermatological problems, or for septic processes (carbuncles, abscesses, etc.), inflammation is reduced and faster healing is promoted.

With these remedies, combined with some of the touch techniques I have discussed in this chapter as developed by Dr Allan, she was soon back to normal and today she is very happy and healthy.

Then there was a very unusual case of a boy who fell on the ice. He had a very nasty fall and damaged his coccyx very badly. After that he lost the sense of touch in several parts of his body. I decided to treat his coccyx as I felt that he described his problems exactly. As the coccyx ends in three small crystals it is very tender. I decided on a treatment method that was rather extreme, but involved energising the coccyx or the ganglion of impar. The main aim of this procedure is to relax any tension in the rectal area (the coccyx). The feet and heel area were tested for the coccyx, and tenderness was elicited. This area has a direct bearing on the prostate in men and the ovaries in women. I positioned him face down and checked for soreness in the reflex areas of the feet (anus). I then stood at the foot of the patient and touched the right side with my right fingers, and on the left with my left fingers. Strange as it may seem, this inner-heel contact will release tension and allow the healing energy to take over.

Another method of this application is to ask patients to bend the knees so that the leg is at right angles, then lift the leg by the ankle and allow it to drop (onto a cushion) with the right hand around the right ankle and the left hand around the left ankle. This has a relaxing effect on the coccyx (impar) area.

This is an extreme treatment and not often practised but in this patient's case I thought it would help. Indeed, when I was able to lift the coccyx very gently, the energy flow came back and much of his feeling was restored. I gave him the homoeopathic remedy *Arnica* and Emergency Essence. To build him up, I gave him Health Insurance Plus from Nature's Best (one capsule a day), and luckily he too completely recovered.

The next case was a man in his mid-forties, who suffered from writer's cramp. This was a major problem for him as he was unable to write or even sign his name. He did nothing about it when the first signs appeared. Then he went to his doctor, and took pills and remedies to no avail. The poor man became frustrated and nervous about his condition. When he came to see me I examined him and saw that he had some neck problems so I gave him electro-acupuncture, some gentle manipulation and prescribed a tablet of ArMax twice a day. This is a marvellous remedy which I have prescribed for a number of years. It is an American remedy which contains key nutrients for the joints such as vitamin C, niacin, pantothenic acid, magnesium, manganese, zinc and boron. ArMax provides these essential nutrients together with a special ingredient called glucosamine sulphate, which is naturally present in joint cartilage. It is a remedy from the Enzymatic Therapy range and can be obtained in this country. He improved after that treatment, so later on we used physiotherapy and he is now able to write again without any effort or discomfort.

A lady aged about seventy suddenly developed a tendency to shake after she experienced an electric shock. She had been changing a light bulb without first turning off the power when the bulb broke. A few weeks after the electric shock she started to shake so badly that she could not even hold a spoon. She was crying as she told me how sorry she felt for her husband, who now had to do everything. I treated her with a remedy called Hyperiforce, as she was so depressed. This remedy contains St John's wort, which is very helpful in such cases. Not only is Hyperiforce beneficial for the nervous system, but it is of great help for the circulatory system. I also gave her a homoeopathic remedy called *Cerebellum*. With these remedies she began to improve, and although she is not yet completely better, she has improved so much that she can again do her share of the housework.

There are many cases in which either the sensory nerves or the motor nerves have been damaged or influenced to the extent that patients lose their sense of touch. There are also many ways to restore touch and although not all cases are successful, people should not believe that problems cannot be overcome and that they have to live with them. Like the little bird and the baby I described at the beginning of this chapter it is always good to remember that positive looks for negative and whatever treatment is used – alternative or orthodox – it helps to keep a positive attitude. If the little bird had enough sense to be aware of the situation, so must we. We must face our problems as soon as they become apparent. When there is something wrong with the body we must set about restoring harmony.

2

Smell

Have you ever had the experience of seeing a beautifully prepared meal with the finest aroma; your mouth is watering, and yet you cannot smell? What a terrible experience! I see many people who complain that they have lost their sense of smell. There are numerous reasons why this might occur. The endocrine system is very finely tuned and needs to work in harmony, otherwise the sense of smell can be affected and we do not smell things as we did before.

This is very often a question of breathing. When I see how people breathe – and sometimes so badly – I say to myself that this must have an effect on the sense organs. Why was I so certain that my little granddaughter Gemma would stay alive? Because I could see she had God-given breathing – in and out of her stomach, quite harmonious, in tune with herself – a newly born creation. It brings me back to what I once wrote in an article: that God took to himself the dust of the earth and from it he made man. He then breathed into his nostrils the breath of life and man became a living soul. It is very important that our capacity to breathe and to smell is as perfect as it can be. They are two functions in life that we desperately need.

When I do a facial diagnosis and I see a person is ill, I look to see what has gone wrong both inside and outside. By observing the way people breathe I know whether their lungs are functioning properly. I can also see how important it is that incorrect breathing is put right. In many of my books I have mentioned the Hara breathing method. In *Stress and Nervous Disorders* I emphasise how important it is to improve our breathing. I hope in this chapter to discuss a few ideas which can help us to smell and breathe in order to enjoy life more. As we grow older it is so easy to miss out on that part in life without realising that there are many ways that we can improve on it, but man seems to be the only creature who is unaware of what he is doing or where he is going. The ants and the bees have advanced knowledge of the part they are destined to play in life.

We lack in-depth knowledge of the physiology of the nervous system and how the mind is influenced by the state of the organs. Leave it to man to get his priorities wrong. Yet mystical laws were in existence long before those of physiology. There is a reason for the slow progress of knowledge of ourselves. Our original way of life within small groups has been replaced by the herd instinct; solitude is now frequently looked upon as a punishment – or sometimes as a luxury. Modern civilisation seems incapable of producing people endowed with imagination, intelligence and courage. Discoveries are developed without any realisation of their consequences. In fact, man is becoming a stranger in his own world.

There is a possible remedy for this evil and it rests in a more profound knowledge of ourselves. The science of man has become the most necessary of all sciences: 'Man is a being composed of matter and consciousness'. Such a proposition is really meaningless. Everybody is animated by an invisible power and this makes the body possess the qualities of a magnet. It is of no ultimate use for us to increase the comfort, the luxury, the beauty and the complications of our civilisation. All this will prove of no value if our weaknesses prevent us using this knowledge to our best advantage. The science of man will, and must be, the task of the future. The soul and body are creations of our methods of observation. The human body is far too complex for us to comprehend in its entirety. The quality of any individual partly depends on that of his surface, as the brain is continually being moulded by the messages it receives from the outside world.

It is necessary for all of us to acknowledge the value of the doctrine; 'Man know thyself'. Ancient mystics believed in this doctrine and proved it in their work. They taught their disciples how to control the vibrations of the pituitary and pineal glands, the glands of the sixth and seventh senses, in a manner that enabled them to contact any region of the inner worlds that they desired to visit, as we do in our dreams as we sleep. This faculty is under the control of the will. It is not necessary for us to go into a trance or do anything abnormal to raise the objective mind to the super-conscious state.

In my youth I spent much of my free time in the family pharmacy and I was often told that I had an exceptional sense of smell. I was told I should go to Paris to create perfumes. My sense of smell and quality of breathing have deteriorated over the years, possibly because of the many plane journeys I have made. When breathing capacity is reduced and body energies go out of balance, we have to pay extra attention to deeper breathing, as well as doing exercises. Practise breathing exercises in the fresh air by exhaling and inhaling in a regular pattern. Breathe deeply when walking or sitting, when you eat or drink, and when you walk or play. Concentrating on breathing properly improves oxygenation and helps the blood circulation.

As breathing means life it cannot be treated superficially. Breathing exercises are important and will be of tremendous help in regaining a sense of smell. Inhale through the nostrils as often as possible. Keep the muscles of your face perfectly relaxed and your mouth closed. Inhale as deeply as possible, avoiding any effort or strain. Correct the position of the chest and keep the spinal column erect. Fill the lungs with air, raise the arms in a sideways circular motion and as high as you can without strain. Then move the tongue, smack the lips, swallow the saliva that has accumulated and, just before exhaling, bring the arms down and throw them behind you. Begin to exhale slowly, emptying the lungs completely.

Repeat this exercise at least seven times. When you have gone through this exercise once you will make a point of doing it regularly, just as enthusiastically as you do the Hara breathing exercise.

Always ensure, when doing breathing exercises, that the lungs are completely emptied. Begin by taking short breaths, one breath in, one breath out, in and out, doing it in different postures, either sitting, kneeling or standing. If you are not successful at first, look for the help of a good teacher, either a singing teacher or someone who specialises in breathing exercises. Never a day passes when I do not do Hara breathing exercises myself, thus gaining the energy required to do my daily work, and I have no doubt that these exercises improve my sense of smell.

When the breathing becomes impaired it is time to take action. I have been very encouraged by the results of aromatherapy and reflexology in such cases. The essential oils used in aromatherapy are highly beneficial. Aromatherapy is a fine therapeutic treatment when combined with massage and touch therapy and when the correct oils are used. The ancient Greeks and Romans used the medical knowledge of the Egyptians, and we have only just begun to discover the value of these traditions.

AROMATHERAPY

Essential oils have been used for centuries and in their pure form they can treat the body as a whole. Essential oils are not fatty – some are even light – but they vary considerably in odour. Some evaporate more quickly than others but they all do a specific job. Above all, the purity of the oil is vitally important.

A penetrating aroma which cultivates all the senses can probably relieve deafness or titillate the taste buds, so that any blockage or obstruction will be overcome. Absorption in the bloodstream is important. Vapourising and inhaling essential oils can be very useful for treating infections. They can also be used in compresses or in a bath and, of course, with massage. Inhaling essential oils combined with breathing exercises can relieve the symptoms of asthma, bronchitis or shortness of breath.

A skilled aromatherapist knows when a particular treatment will be effective. An unskilled aromatherapist, however, may use oils which can damage a patient. I have great admiration for Shirley Price, Tisserand, Body Oils and other companies which have done so much to develop this wonderful therapy. When I worked with Mrs Lubinic in Heidelberg, Germany, I found that she used only the purest oils and with her I developed a range of oils that have since been used successfully by aromatherapists in conjunction with the essential flower essences. It is wonderful to see how geranium oil can change a mood almost instantly, how tea tree oil can clear an attack of cystitis, or how jasmine can be so helpful for depression. A heavy menstrual period can be relieved with chamomile and a cold with eucalyptus. There is much to be learned from books on aromatherapy. Parts of that wonderful sense of smell can be very quickly triggered by an essential oil. The memory centres can play a role in the emotional response once an odour is inhaled, and it is interesting to learn the olfactory epithelium contains more than twenty million nerve endings.

The hypothalamus, which receives the message, acts immediately and sends messages to the other part of the brain. In my previous book, *How to Live a Healthy Life*, I referred many times to the fact that man has three bodies: a physical, mental and emotional body. Since the influence of odour has such a tremendous ability to affect our emotions, aromatherapy almost shouts that we should give it a place in today's medicine. We have to see these three bodies as a whole and when treating a single sense we should take all five senses into account. When working in the garden, especially if we have not used artificial fertilisers, we experience how evocative the scents of honeysuckle or newly mown grass can be. In the oldest book, the Bible, we can read in the Song of Solomon about pleasant fruits and spices such as saffron, cinnamon, spikenard, myrrh and aloe. Such references also occur in the New Testament, where we read of the precious oils that were used for healing. In Psalm 104 we read that God gave man a promise that He would cause the grass to grow for the cattle, but a herb for the service of man. Even now, in this day and age, this promise is fulfilled. Essential oils are the vital elements of plants, often considered the vegetable hormones. They can be taken from various different parts of the plants. Unfortunately, true essential oils are not always readily available.

My great friend, Jo Serrentino, with whom I worked for Dr Vogel, has studied essential oils for many years. She has observed that essential oils are a complex formula of organic chemicals naturally produced by the plant. The life and growing conditions of the plant are all imprinted in the characteristics of the essential oil. Such an oil can contain as many as two hundred organic chemicals; for example, essential oil of rosemary, having a high concentration of the oxide 1.8 sineol, acts as a mucolytic breaking down mucus and targets the respiratory system, whereas an oil with a high concentration of the ketone verbanone has a strong cleansing effect on the liver.

In my book *Body Energy* I have emphasised the potential health properties of essential oils. Much of the responsibility for our health rests on our own shoulders and it is in our best interests to pay attention to any indicators. I often remind patients of the words of Dr Osler, a man with an admirable medical background: when the nerves of the eyes and feet are properly understood, there will be less need for surgical intervention.

You may know that karate is a Japanese system of self-defence, but perhaps you do not know the origin of the word: *kara* means open, and *te* means hand. Therefore karate means 'open hand'. You may wonder why I refer to karate in a book on energy and ways of balancing the body for the maintenance of good health. This is because true karate is a martial art which is concerned with the balance of the mind and body in *defence*; it is never to be used in *attack*. True health is also the balancing of the mind and body in defence, against attack from bacteria and other harmful influences from the outside.

All natural therapies aim to keep the body in balance, naturally endeavouring to maintain harmony between the different bodily systems – and the mind. When you correct an imbalance, good health will prevail once more. Most people tend to want others to take responsibility for maintaining their health, when in fact the balance is restored more quickly when patients themselves take an active and therefore positive part in their recovery, both physically and mentally. The prime responsibility must always be with the patient, helped by expert guidance from the therapist. In the case of aromatherapy treatments, it is advisable for therapists to give the client 'homework' in one or both of the following forms:

- pure oils to inhale and/or add to the bath
- mixed oils or lotions to apply to the face and/or body, not only to help the cause of the problem, but also to alleviate the symptoms that are visible and therefore upsetting to the patient.

The body has its own natural in-built ability to heal itself, but when it does need help, natural therapies together with a positive approach on the part of both therapist and patient can usually do the job without resorting to synthetic pills and tablets with their accompanying side-effects.

An interesting test was recently conducted in the field of conventional medicine. A group of people with the same problem were equally divided into two halves. One half saw a consultant who gave them positive encouragement, showed real interest in their problems, and gave them a positive diagnosis and an optimistic forecast. The consultant for the second half had a more negative and disinterested approach. I don't need to tell you that a much higher rate of recovery was evident among the people in the first group.

During consultations (and this is so for all complementary therapists with whom I have come into contact), it always pays to get the patient actively involved. Aromatherapists, unless they have other specialised training, are not usually qualified to make a diagnosis. Trained people use the reflexes of the feet and ask relevant questions to discover both the physical and mental state of the patient and, of course, they spend time listening, so that the emotional state of the whole person can be assessed. From the answers they are given, it is possible to deduce which oils are most likely to revitalise the systems of the body which are out of balance.

Aromatherapy means the use of aromas from essential oils to therapeutically revitalise and strengthen the cellular tissues. It should be stressed that I am talking of *essential oils* here, as nowadays a few people trade in 'aromatherapy oils', which are not always pure and unadulterated.

Only true essential oils which have been either distilled or expressed from the plant of the same name (nothing is added and nothing is taken away) are used in true aromatherapy. The exceptions are two well-known absolutes, rose and jasmine (very expensive) and benzoin resin (quite expensive). These three are not pure essential oils, as solvents are used in the extraction process, but they are used by most professional aromatherapists in mixes for application to the skin or use in the bath. They should never be used internally.

Each essential oil has the ability to help improve one or more systems within the body, and many of the oils help to reduce what is commonly known as stress, in day-to-day living, or depression, which can occur as the result of anxiety or stressful events.

Essential oils (like many other forms of complementary medicine) can restore energy, balance and harmony to a person's body rhythm when this has been interrupted by what is popularly called disease, i.e. they help to restore ease where there is dis-ease.

They can effect an improvement by themselves, for example when a person uses them in a simple home treatment in a fragrant bath for relaxation, following the guidance of a therapist or a specialist aromatherapy book. They can also be used in conjunction with many other complementary therapies such as osteopathy, acupuncture, remedial massage or skin treatments.

How is the use of essential oils different from using the whole plant? To answer that we need to know where the essential oil is to be found, and also to realise that its power is highly concentrated. One drop of essential oil in 5 ml (a teaspoonful) of vegetable oil is sufficient to give the characteristic aroma of the plant.

Apart from expressed volatile oils, all of which are found in the skins of citrus fruits, essential oils can be found in the petals, leaves, seeds, stems, bark and roots of various plants, bushes or trees. They are present in very small amounts, locked in tiny oil 'glands' which burst during distillation to release their precious oil.

When the whole plant is used, the concentration of healing power is necessarily spread over a greater area, so more plant material is needed to produce a similar result. Also, plants hold other healing properties in their structure which are made use of in herbal medicine. Aromatherapists use only the essential oils, which have quite a few advantages.

- They take up less space, so are much more convenient for travelling and holidays.
- They are ready for instant use, and will keep more or less indefinitely. The therapeutic qualities of some whole plants can change drastically after being stored for some time.
- The therapeutic effect is considerably magnified in the essential oil compared to the whole plant.
- They can be used in a greater variety of ways.

It is important to know that some plants contain more essential oil than others, so the cost of essential oils varies immensely. It is also important to know that a true essential oil, without adulteration of any kind, is of necessity more expensive than an oil of the same name which has been 'standardised', i.e. given a British pharmaceutical standard, which may even mean that alterations have been made to the natural oil to enable it to conform to what can be a lower standard than many plants are capable of producing.

When selecting oils the most important points for a therapist to remember are as follows:

- No harmful chemical fertilisers or pesticides should have been used in their production (including those that produce quick lush growth, because just as forced strawberries have no flavour, the resulting oil is of a poorer quality).
- Oils should be chosen without the addition of alcohol, nature-identical components, synthetic smell-alikes, or cheaper natural oils.

Pure essential oils are magical! Their power is such that they should not be used in their concentrated form on the skin. There are a few exceptions to this rule, for example when treating burns and insect bites and other specific instances. In all other cases essential oils are always used in a carrier of some sort, i.e. anything neutral which carries the essential oil into the body.

A prime example of such a carrier is air, which carries essential oils into our noses when we inhale from a tissue. In fact, inhalation is one of the best ways, if not the best way, of using essential oils. Because our nasal passages have a direct line of contact with the brain, undiluted essential oils are put to work almost immediately to relieve problems like sudden stress, depression, headaches, respiratory disorders and insomnia.

Some of the oils which help such conditions are listed below:

Sudden stress: basil, juniper, lavender, cedarwood, neroli, rose.
Depression: basil, bergamot, clary-sage, thyme, chamomile,
                  camphor, geranium, lavender, frankincense, jasmine,
                  neroli, patchouli, rose, sandalwood, ylang-ylang.
Headaches: lemon, eucalyptus, aniseed, chamomile, lavender.
Asthma: basil, cajuput, lemon, sage, thyme, aniseed, cypress,
                  hyssop, lavender, marjoram, melissa, peppermint, pine,
                  rosemary, savory, benzoin, clove, origanum.
Sinus problems: basil, eucalyptus, lemon, neroli, lavender, peppermint,
                  pine, clove.
Insomnia: basil, chamomile, camphor, juniper, lavender, marjoram,
                  neroli, rose, sandalwood, ylang-ylang.

Water is also a very useful carrier, especially when the oils are added to a warm bath. For all the above complaints (except asthma, as the hot water makes the oils evaporate too quickly and they are then too powerful for an asthmatic to cope with), plus general aches and pains, poor circulation, ongoing stress, period problems, certain skin conditions and sore throats, six to eight drops of the appropriate essential oils in the bath will produce amazing results in most cases.

Some oils that will help these additional conditions are listed below:

Aches and pains: cajuput, coriander, caraway, eucalyptus, sage, thyme,
                 black pepper, chamomile, camphor, juniper, lavender,

	marjoram, rosemary, clove, ginger, nutmeg, origanum.
Poor circulation:	lemon, black pepper, camphor, cypress, juniper, rosemary, benzoin, rose, ginger.
Ongoing stress:	basil, bergamot, clary-sage, petit-grain, thyme, chamomile, geranium, juniper, lavender, marjoram, melissa, benzoin, cedarwood, jasmine, patchouli, rose, sandalwood.
Painful periods:	cajuput, sage, aniseed, chamomile, cypress, juniper, marjoram, melissa, peppermint, rosemary, jasmine, tarragon.
PMT:	lavender, melissa, neroli, rose, geranium, chamomile, clary-sage.
Eczema:	sage, chamomile, hyssop, geranium, lavender, bergamot, juniper, sandalwood.
Sore throat:	eucalyptus, thyme, cajuput, cedarwood, sandalwood, lemon, tea tree.

Gargling is another way in which water can be used as a carrier for these natural oils and is invaluable for treating a sore throat or a cough. Add two or three drops of essential oil to half a cup of warm water and gargle with this to soothe and to kill off the infection (stirring before each mouthful as essential oils do not completely dissolve in water).

This is an appropriate place to make the point that essential oils in any carrier need to be used regularly in order to achieve the desired effect. Moreover, in cases of infection, their use should be continued beyond the 'feeling better' stage, rather like a course of antibiotics, to ensure that the symptoms will not recur.

Compresses, again with water as the carrier, are most effective for localised problems such as arthritis, period problems, ulcers, athlete's foot, sprains and bruises; and for a bad head cold or catarrh sinuses inhaling from a bowl of hot water and essential oils clears the head in minutes. (Remember, however, in cases of asthma hot water should not be used with essential oils.)

The last way of using essential oils with water as the carrier is, I think, an excellent one. It is possible to make tea using essential oils. If possible, tannin-free teabags should be used, though ordinary ones will do to make a very weak basic brew. If you have a stomach upset you may choose to put two drops of peppermint and one drop of fennel onto a teabag over which you pour one and a half pints of nearly boiling water. Stir well and remove the teabag. Then drink one cup of tea three times a day, saving the rest in a jug in the fridge until it is needed again.

It is great fun to make teas to help you sleep, teas to relieve stress, teas for reviving your brain (if you have a lot of work to do) and all from one box of teabags and a few little bottles!

One of the most popular methods of using essential oils is by application to the skin. Professional aromatherapists use a vegetable oil as a carrier so that they can carry out the special massage techniques now associated with aromatherapy. Shiatsu pressures, lymph drainage, neuro-muscular massage together with effleurage movements make up this form of massage, and it is one of the best and most pleasurable treatments that exist for dealing with stress and its associated problems.

A well-trained aromatherapist will mix you a bottle of the oils that have been used in your treatment for your own use at home. You may be given them in their pure form for inhalation, baths or teas and perhaps also in a carrier oil or non-greasy lotion (the latter is much more pleasant to apply) for use after your bath or shower.

The skin responds very well to the application of essential oils in carrier oils, lotions or creams. A good quality aromatherapy skin-care range will rejuvenate the skin when used regularly, softening and smoothing its texture. People with problem skins, blocked sinuses, eczema, headaches, etc. can, with a specially formulated aromatherapy moisturising cream, take care of their skin at the same time as treating these problems. A hand lotion especially developed for arthritis softens the skin while at the same time relieving pain and making movement easier.

A new aromatherapy treatment developed by Shirley Price, called Swiss Reflex Therapy, is very similar to reflexology. It is now practised by quite a few aromatherapists, using essential oils. The patient takes an active part in the treatment, and is shown how to continue this at home, which may explain why it is proving so successful.

Swiss Reflex Therapy can be used in combination with an aromatherapy massage of the part of the body involved, or on its own where a massage would be difficult, contra-indicated or unhelpful, for example if the part were swollen and painful. All the work on the feet is carried out to the pain threshold of each individual and the improvement is monitored by the patients themselves.

Aromatherapy is an amazing, delightful and rewarding therapy which fills anyone who embarks upon its study with never-ending enthusiasm. Because it is still in its infancy, being relatively new to this country, new facts are being discovered every day, and more research and attention is being given to the quality and the content of the essential oils used. Courses in aromatherapy are already getting longer, in order to accommodate the increasing amount of theory which needs to be taught. One day, no doubt, it will be necessary to take a degree in something or other in order to practise aromatherapy. However, that may prevent many caring people from being able to take it up as a career and doing useful work to help the lives of themselves and others. The aspect which must not suffer in this thirst for more theoretical knowledge is the practical application; this must remain of prime importance, I believe, as aromatherapy is probably the only therapy which can be carried out in its simplest form by anyone and everyone who first steps onto this fascinating path for restoring energy.

The immune system, which is our body's defence against infections, functions with the support of the lymph system. Nowadays I see many cases of lymphatic congestion where the body's immune system is not aided in the defence it needs. Much toxic waste material is stored in the lymph system and affects the mental and emotional state of the individual. This can lead to very serious illnesses such as ME (myalgic encephalomyelitis), post-viral fatigue syndrome or other problems. Essential oils are a powerful support for the immune system and play an important role in preventing infections. Illness, either chronic or temporary, changes our sense of smell because of influences constantly affecting the odour stimuli.

One of my greatest worries is that over the years pollution of the air, water and soil has led the plant fibre to thicken and become weaker in colour. We see a nutritionally degenerative plant and yet when we remove the oil we find the same strong vital force in the chemistry – as strong as it was one thousand years ago. It is wonderful to see the immunity of plants where the oil still carries the life force and therefore has the ability to regenerate and protect life in itself. The 'intelligence' within essential oils is a great tool with which to reach the deep recesses of our brain and cross over the chemical barriers.

It is wonderful to see today that this great gift to mankind is still of the greatest importance. I used to do occasional spells of voluntary work in the Open Air Bible Museum in the Netherlands and I took the opportunity to study the ancient civilisations. It was then I learned how the Egyptians were the first to discover the potentials of fragrance. According to records dating back to 4500 BC, balsamic substances with aromatic properties were used for religious rituals, and also in medicine. When King Tut's tomb was opened in 1922, 350 litres of oils were discovered in alabaster jars. The ancient Egyptians and the Babylonians believed that in order to reach a higher level they had to be clean, as was also the case in Roman and Arab civilisations. Later, during the thirteenth and fourteenth centuries essential oils were considered so valuable that they were often stolen. Numerous references can be found in the Bible to the value of oils, from the Creation right up to the time of Christ.

During one of my lecture tours in the United States, I met a very fine aromatherapist from North Carolina. She attended one of my lectures and afterwards she asked me which oil was best to heal scar tissue. Without hesitation I replied that it was St John's wort. In my London clinic, I see a number of people who, as a result of fire or accidents, have been left badly scarred. I do cosmetic acupuncture for these people, always using St John's wort oil for healing.

Gary Young, who is a naturopath, said that essential oils are a missing link in modern health philosophies, and that they have a bio-electrical energy that is constantly between any two points. Although everything has an electrical frequency, essential oils have a much greater frequency than herbs and foods.

The applications and use of essential oils

MASSAGE

The concept of individuality is important in aromatherapy and it is rare for two people to react in exactly the same way. Massage encourages circulation and eases minor aches and pains. It enables the essential oils to be absorbed and used by the skin and body.

Choose a vegetable-based carrier oil (the following are usually used in aromatherapy):

Grapeseed oil	Avocado oil
Peachnut oil	Calendula oil
Almond oil	Evening Primrose oil
Hypericum oil	

The dosage should be as follows:

Adults: 12 drops essential oil to 50 ml carrier oil
Children (7–14 years): 6 drops essential oil to 50 ml carrier oil
Children (2–7 years): 3 drops essential oil to 50 ml carrier oil
Babies: 1 drop essential oil to 50 ml carrier oil

Given below are guidelines for an aromatherapy massage.

Abdomen

- Apply enough oil to the abdominal area and rub in with effleurage movements. Begin with the hands overlapping, effleurage down to the side and lift and bring downwards toward the pelvis and begin again. (Repeat 4–6 times.)
- Bring the hands to the starting position. Reinforce a diamond following the inside bones of the rib cage and pelvis. Finish below the navel. (Repeat 4–6 times.)
- Keep the hands reinforced, using the palms of the hands only, go clockwise in a circular movement. (Once only.)
- Keep the hands overlapped below the navel for one minute, with the

centre palm over this point.

- Apply stroking movements on the abdomen with the palms and fingers following the direction of the colon. Begin at first on the left side of the colon. (Repeat 6–10 times on each side.)
- Start with the heels of the hands at the navel and push the fingers and heels down to the side. Do this only on soft parts of the abdomen. (Repeat 4–6 times.)
- Aeroplane moment. Push alternate hands toward the top of diamond, using the entire hand. (Repeat 4–6 times.)

Back

- Lying face down give a spinal stretch once, keeping the arms straight. Apply oil.
- Stand at the head of the bed and give reverse effleurage down the centre back lightly, and up the sides of body to the armpits with pressure. Think palm. (Repeat 4–5 times.) Hands begin with the fir tree shape (to cover more of the client's back and the fingers open round the buttocks and come up the sides of body still open. The palms of hands should be down on body to the wrist during the whole of this movement. On the last upward stroke lift the 'head' hand (hand nearest the client's head) off the body as you reach armpit level. Without a break in continuity, turn the 'foot' hand (hand nearest the client's feet) on the body as you walk round to the right side of the client, turning the hand so that the fingertips face the left shoulder. Reinforce with the head hand.
- Give firm effleurage in a figure of eight over the shoulder blades. Think palm. (Repeat 4–5 times.) Move through the shoulder blades in an upward direction and around the left shoulder with palm pressure. Relax on the downward part of the movement, taking the hands upward towards the right shoulder with palm pressure. Relax on the downward stroke and repeat in a continuous figure of eight. Finish by taking each hand to the appropriate shoulder.
- Apply thumb circles around the shoulders. (Repeat 4–5 times.) Lift up the palms, leaving the fingers as an anchor at shoulder level. Circle around the shoulder area with thumb friction and return lightly with the whole hand to base of spine.
- Effleurage over whole back, with fir tree hands and palms right down.

Think palm. (Repeat 4–5 times.) Apply pressure with the palms on the upward movement round the shoulder blades, and a gentle return down sides of body. Finish at the waist with the thumbs either side of spine.

- Apply deep thumb pressures circling along the lumbar and sacral nerve pathways. Make four rainbow archways in all, getting progressively smaller. The first is at waist level, starting with the thumbs in the spinal channel. The thumb friction is done within a one-inch (2.5 cm) diameter, moving out along the top of the iliac crest and down the sides of the buttocks. Lift the thumbs and return with the fingers, placing the thumbs down one inch lower than the first arch. Repeat twice more, each arch being one inch lower than, and inside, the previous one. The last arch is just around the sacrum.

- Fan effleurage up each side of the back, with pressure on the side of hand nearest the spine. Start with the foot hand on the side of body nearest to you, at the base of the spine. Push up with the whole hand, keeping the fingers facing towards the head all the time and the ulnar border going up the spinal channel (for two hands' length). Swing out to the side of body, opening the fingers, and as you do this bring the head hand under the first one at that level and push up for two hands' length with the whole palm, but this time the index finger goes up the spinal channel. Swing out to the side of body, opening the fingers, and bring the foot hand under fanning hand and begin again; 6–8 strokes are all that is needed to ensure the last stroke being done round the shoulder blades with the head hand. This enables the strokes to start again with the foot hand at the base of the spine. Do 3–4 rows of 6–8 strokes, before repeating on the other side of the back.

- Take care this time to keep the ulnar border of the head hand and index finger of the foot hand going up the spinal column on the upward part of stroke. Finish with the head hand so that the foot hand can be straight to the buttock crease as though to repeat another fan – but instead it is ready for the next movement and is joined by head hand (both hands together make a wide 'W').

- Push up from the buttocks to the waist with the thumbs and out to the sides with pressure, using the thenar muscle. (Repeat 4–5 times.) With length of the thumb and thenar muscle giving pressure, push up to and past the waist level until the thenar muscle is sitting in the waist. Swing thumb to index finger, turn the fingers towards the sides of the body until the tips touch the bed, then, as they bend, continue the movement firmly with the thenar muscle across the waist and onto the bed, making a fist.

BATHING

Bathing with essential oils is not just a pleasant way to relax, it can help to relieve many aches and pains and other physical conditions. Add a maximum of 6–7 drops of pure essential oil to your bath (with the water not too hot, approximately 30º C). This proportion is for a healthy adult; for children, 2–3 drops of essential oil will be sufficient, and for babies, 1 drop (it may be mixed with carrier oil or milk, especially if the baby has sensitive skin).

Stir the water well to disperse the oils. Do not use any other bath oils, salts or foam preparations at the same time. Close the windows and doors and relax for 10–20 minutes. You will benefit from the action of the oil, both on your skin and in the water vapour.

SOME USEFUL ADVICE ON AROMATHERAPY

The following notes of caution are taken from *Aromatherapy for the Family*, a booklet published by the Institute of Classical Aromatherapy.

- Aromatherapy can be very helpful during pregnancy and labour, but only under qualified guidance; if you are pregnant, you are strongly advised to consult a qualified aromatherapist.
- Some oils are stimulants, which may sometimes affect people suffering from epilepsy. Sufferers should seek medical advice before using essential oils.
- For babies and small children, use extra diluted quantities.
- Keep bottles out of reach of small children.
- Unless specially indicated, do not apply neat oils directly onto the skin, as they can cause irritation.
- For the same reason, it is advisable to give yourself a patch test on a small area of the skin when using your own blend. Note that certain drugs, stress, and the menstrual cycle can also affect your sensitivity.
- Keep oils away from the eyes, and do not rub your eyes after handling. If you should get any in your eyes, wash them out with plenty of cold water; seek medical advice if necessary.

- Essential oils are flammable, so do not put them on or near a naked flame.
- Some oils are solvents and may damage certain plastics and polished wood surfaces.
- Never take them by mouth, unless under medical instruction.
- If you are taking homoeopathic remedies, check with your practitioner before using essential oils, as it is believed that strong aromas can cancel the effects of homoeopathic medicine.
- If you suffer from skin or other allergies, use the oils very carefully, and patch test before using widely. If you are unfortunate enough to have an allergic reaction to perfume, you are likely to be allergic to some essential oils. In this case, seek some other, gentler form of therapy, such as homoeopathy or the Bach Flower Remedies.
- If in any doubt at all, consult a qualified aromatherapist.

The advice below is reproduced from the 'Buyer's Guide to Aromatherapy Products' in the excellent magazine *Here's Health*, which appears monthly and provides much useful guidance.

- Smell is probably the best guide from both a subjective and an objective point of view, but it is sometimes difficult for the untrained nose to distinguish between a pure essential oil and other fragrances. Nevertheless, if it smells synthetic, don't buy it.
- Don't buy cheap brands. Essential oils are more expensive than synthetic fragrances, and pure essential oils of rose, jasmine, neroli, sandalwood, melissa and German chamomile are particularly dear. Generally, the higher the percentage of oil used, the higher the price.
- Read the label. If oil percentages are not given, look at where they appear in the contents list. Ingredients will have to be listed in descending order of volume/weight as of January 1997; many manufacturers already use this system.
- Remember that botanical names can refer to either essential oils or herb extracts.
- Be wary of products containing fragrance or perfume, particularly if they appear near the top of the ingredients list.
- Avoid products containing mineral oil.

BACH FLOWER REMEDIES

For many years I have been a great admirer of Dr Edward Bach and I have promoted the Bach Flower Remedies in many radio and television programmes. Since I started writing my first book, in the 1980s, I have emphasised the fact that every plant, every leaf and every root has a message. As long as we learn to recognise the message and to see the characteristics and signatures of plants and flowers, we will be able to use them to help ourselves.

In the 1930s, when Dr Bach promoted his views on flower remedies, he was often misunderstood. Today, in the late 1990s, we have totally different problems. I decided to take a fresh look at the healing potential of flowers and I felt a new approach was needed, resulting in a new product called Emergency Essence. I felt that Emergency Essence could probably make a valuable contribution toward dealing with today's emotional problems. One of the main ingredients in Emergency Essence is chamomile, which helps to maintain the equilibrium of mood and mind, and provides relief in acute situations of trauma and emotional upsets. As well as chamomile, this essence includes lavender, red clover, purple coneflower, self-heal and yarrow. I have received letters from all over the world, remarking on the beneficial results people have obtained using this essence.

As I have said many times in my books, Nature cures and in Nature everything is in balance. Imbalance is caused by man. These flower essences have been of tremendous help in many awkward situations. The widespread interest in Emergency Essence encouraged me to look further into the compositions of herbs and flowers.

Flower essences are liquid extracts of flowers in a base of grape alcohol. They can be taken orally and are believed to influence feelings of emotional well-being. In turn they may have an impact on the health of the whole body. Although flowers have been used in healthcare for many centuries, the use of flower essences to influence specific emotions and attitudes was developed and refined in Britain in the 1930s. Since then, essences have gained increasing recognition all over the world for their significant contribution to holistic healthcare. Today, essences are made from flowers obtained from all corners of the globe; many species of plants may only be found in areas such as the Australian bush, Californian desert and Israel.

The characteristics of many of these plants have now been described, and they provide us with essences possessing unique properties. My mind at this moment goes back to Dr Bach, who saw the language of flowers, plants and herbs and, like myself, looked at their characteristics. Nature does not lie and it will give us its signatures. You do not need to spend long looking at the *Gingko biloba* and the form of its leaves to see how they resemble the human brain. The two leaves hang by a little stem, positive and negative, but yet holistically held together. In the previous chapter we discussed how negative and positive should be in harmony.

If we look at a leaf of St John's wort under a microscope, we see thousands of minute holes, surrounded by that wonderful healing oil. This plant is named after the apostle St John. In all the different essences that Dr Bach tried out he found a solution. I was once told that Dr Bach was inspired by an old book, over one hundred years old, called *The Language of Flowers*. Some time ago I came across a copy in an antique shop. It was old and falling to bits, but the message is as clear today as it ever was. In the introduction the writer of this book, who is not named, says that 'when we look at the language and poetry of flowers, we look at the gift to the young and sensitive or to all ages, rejoicing in what nature has to offer'. The book contains poems about many flowers, ranging from dandelions to chamomile. Even the primrose is mentioned as helping all ills of life. Hundreds of plants, flowers and herbs are suggested for different problems, for example meadowsweet for inadequacy, mint for virtue, pansy for thought, heath for solitude and the vine for intoxication.

After having read this book, I started to compile the Jan de Vries combination flower essences, because I wanted to share these wonderful combinations with others. These plants, flowers and herbs are a gift from our Creator, who has signed them with characteristics that reveal their use.

If we think of our Creator giving man the promise of the foods to exist and the herbs for healing that are mentioned in the Old Testament, we can see what these essences should be used for:

Female Essence:	she oak, evening primrose, lady's mantle, lavender, mariposa lily.
	To help maintain a feeling of emotional balance and well-being in women. May be chosen around the time of your period.
Bowel Essence:	tormentil, centaury, kapok bush, peppermint, chamomile, yarrow, dandelion.
	To help maintain bowel comfort and function.
Vitality Essence:	caperberry, aloe vera, olive, Siberian ginseng, wild rose, zinnia.
	To help maintain a feeling of motivation and drive. Could help maintain a zest for life, supporting general well-being.
Child Essence:	impatiens, wild oat, black-eyed Susan, mariposa lily, chamomile.
	To help maintain a feeling of calm and restfulness. Could help to maintain a sense of physical and mental well-being.
Male Essence:	agrimony, sequoia, sticky monkey flower, flannel flower, sunflower, dandelion, damiana.
	To help maintain a feeling of physical and emotional well-being in men.
Concentration Essence:	ginkgo, Siberian ginseng, cosmos, madia, rosemary.
	To help maintain a feeling of mental alertness. May be chosen by those who have to deal with many details at once.
Emergency Essence:	chamomile, lavender, red clover, purple coneflower, self-heal, yarrow.
	To help maintain equilibrium of mood and mind. It may be used in acute situations such as emotional upsets.

I have been particularly surprised at the tremendous success of Vitality Essence, especially for older people. Vitality Essence contains caperberry which is mentioned in a very old translation of the book of Ecclesiastes in the Old Testament. These particular flowers, which grow so well in Israel, are found in valleys and on rockeries. The story portrays an allegorical insight into the cycle of life. The writer of Ecclesiastes refers to old age, when a person weakens and body organs break down. Ecclesiastes describes this 'wintertime' of life in symbolic language – as when the sun, moon and stars darken, and the clouds of affliction appear and increase a person's troubles. That is when the light of the sun, the moon and the stars will grow dim for you. Then your arms, that have protected you, will tremble, and your legs, now strong, will grow weak. Your teeth will be too few to chew your food, and your eyes too dim to see clearly. Your ears will be deaf to the noise of the street. You will barely be able to hear the mill as it grinds or music as it plays, not even the song of a bird will wake you from sleep. Your hair will turn white; you will hardly be able to drag yourself along, and all desire will have gone.

The silver chain (spinal cord) will snap, and the golden lamp (brain) will fall and break; the rope at the well will break, and the water jar (heart) shall be shattered.

In the very old translation I refer to, this passage is followed by a reference to the caperberry. 'When the caperberry changes from flowers into berries we have to think and look.' I have found the caperberry to be a valuable constituent of Vitality Essence and the results exceed my expectations.

I had a wonderful time investigating these flower essences, their uses and their tremendous benefits. I enjoyed a visit to the Australian bush, where I was challenged on the flowers. I did not know what was growing in the bush but I could clearly see the benefits by their characteristics and signatures and so I went on to use them in some of my treatments. In his marvellous book *Bush Flower Essences*, Ian White describes many of the bush flowers that have been discovered, and are so helpful, and he refers to them as the 'fruits of the earth'. They have been used for healing by the Aborigines for centuries.

Very often, the secret lies in the composition of the essences. Dr Bach was astute when he made horse chestnut essence from the bud. Flower essences derived from buds are valuable, and many mothers-to-be who have taken the essence of horse chestnut, six weeks prior to giving birth, will bear this out.

Below I give some examples of plant definitions, as described in the old literature:

Chamomile: deeply relaxed and at ease; objective in examining emotions and emotionally at peace.

Nasturtium (a well-known kitchen herb) :
                expresses an earthly nature; alive with vital energy. Nasturtium, nowadays, is a wonderful herb with which to stimulate the endocrine system and balance the thyroid.

Red clover: centred and balanced in the face of emotional hysteria; responds calmly and creatively to crisis and fear of the future. This flower has a calming influence on excitable people.

Sunflower: unique and radiant; high self-esteem; individuality; self-healing. Sunflower seed oil is helpful for harmonising imbalances.

Self-heal: the name is self-explanatory – healing power; confidence; clarity; nourishment. Self-heal is an excellent healer for trauma and similar problems.

Borage: cheerful; confident in the face of danger; uplifting and encouraging.

This form of old medicine still plays a part in medicine today. Let us use it and try to harmonise with our Creator and Nature.

SYMPATHETIC THERAPY

Now let's look at the main causes that impair our sense of smell. The greatest enemy must be congestion. Out of all diseases congestion is a major killer. I never fail to impress on people how essential it is that congestion must be treated. A common cold can easily lead to a bigger problem which will make us lose our sense of smell. I have seen many common colds develop into an infection in the sinuses or the mucous membranes; or the bronchi can be affected as is the case in bronchitis or asthmatic problems.

The minute that the sinuses become affected we have to be especially careful because the sinuses communicate, directly or indirectly, with the nasal cavity. They receive the breath of life directly and unmodified as it flows from the universe through the nose filter, before any other organ has a chance to select and absorb any substance.

The sinuses are lined with a mucous membrane extending from the nose and thus rapidly spread all disorders that affect the nose. The nose is the first organ to react to polluted air and that reaction

Figure 8: Paralysis – tabes

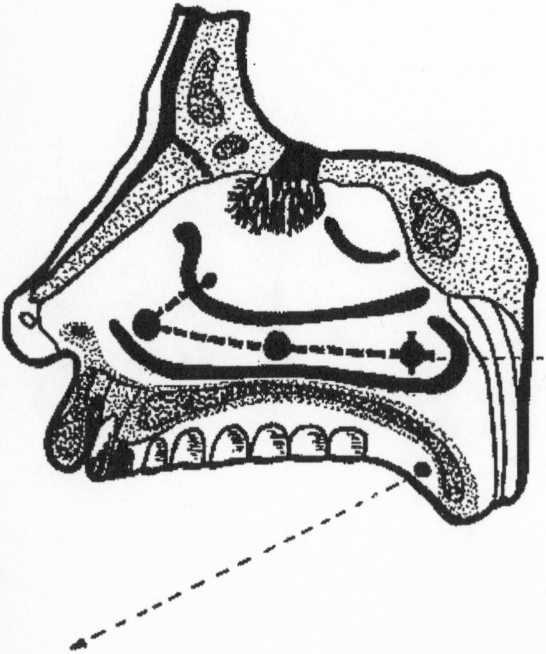

Galvanic

Buccal touch is made above the uvula

Note Touch with a heavy contact. Posterior touch with light galvanic.

is called a cold. The inflammation resulting from the effects of the polluted air extends from the nasal mucous lining to the sinuses, causing such disorders as frontal headache (frontal sinus), pain in the cheek (maxillary sinus), pain between the eyes (ethmoidal sinus) and deep-seated pain in the back of the eyes (sphenoidal sinus). Trouble starts when, in inflammatory conditions, the mucous excretions of the lining of the maxillary sinus fill up as the orifice is at the upper part.

The Sankys Doctrine states that the five physical senses of conscious man are the exteriorised products of the five corresponding spiritual centres. These are as follows:

Figure 9: Sympathetic nasal zones

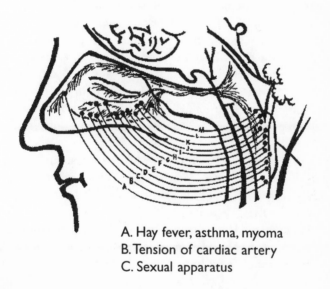

A. Hay fever, asthma, myoma
B. Tension of cardiac artery
C. Sexual apparatus

D. Endocrine
E. Incontinence, bladder
F. Menstruation, pain in hip, sciatica
G. Enteritis, constipation
H. Relaxation of diaphragm

I. Kidney
J. Stomach
K. Liver
L. Ear, dizziness
M. Anguish, anxiety

1. Frontal sinus: a cavity in the frontal bone of the skull.
2. Sphenoidal sinus: a cavity in the sphenoid bone of the skull.
3. Maxillary sinus: the largest of the five, resembling a pyramid in shape.
4. Palatine sinus: a cavity in the orbital process of the palatine bone and opening into either the sphenoidal or posterior ethmoidal sinus.
5. Ethmoidal sinus: this chamber consists of numerous cavities occupying the labyrinth of the ethmoid bone and in these cavities are situated the small mysterious glands known as the intellectual organs.

These sinuses, or air centres, and the small glands within them, constitute the spiritual sense centres that receive a higher intelligence, which is too subtle for contact by the five physical senses of conscious man. Into these chambers or sinuses, there incessantly flows a peculiar gaseous substance, known to the ancients as the mental spirit. The small glands, the intellectual organs, located in the skull near the point where the nose joins the forehead are activated by the mental spirit that passes through the nostrils into the ordinate and collaborate with the sinuses.

Polluted air damages these sinuses and thus the body's ability to resist disease is weakened and the power to attain intuitive powers is also diminished. These chambers are in direct contact with the pineal and pituitary glands, and are also part of the universal mind.

Figure 10 shows a good example of what is known as reflex action, where the essential elements are a nervous centre, a nerve conveying ingoing impulses (afferent nerve) and a nerve conveying outgoing impulses (efferent nerve).

The anterior (front) representation of the sympathetic nervous system starts at the Scheiderian membrane in the nose and ends in the rectum (ganglion of impar) and the perineum. Drs Bonnier and Gillet of France have both produced phenomenal results in cases which had previously been classed as incurable by this stimulation of the positive (nasal) and negative (impar) poles of the body.

Another powerful adjunct is the use of the nasal probe on the mucocutaneous margin in the patient's nose. Always use the probe on the margin toward the outer side of both nostrils. Nasal

NASAL SYMPATHY THROUGH THE MUCOSA

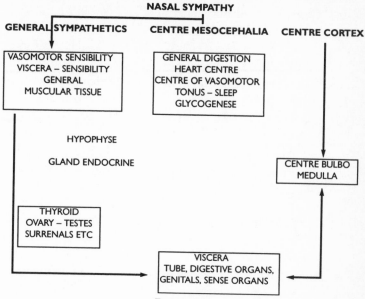

Figure 10

branches of the ophthalmic division of the fifth nerve and nasal branches of the anterior palatine descend from Meckel's ganglion, which is connected with the superior maxillary division of the fifth nerve. This conducts sensory influence to the medulla. There it is reflexed to the respiratory, pneumogastric and other centres. Nerves of the nasal fossa are nasal branches of the ophthalmic to the septum and connect anterior branches of the superior maxillary to the inferior turbinate and the floor of the nose.

The spheno-palatine ganglion gives off the vidian nerve to the septum and superior turbinate. The superior nasal branch goes to the naso-palatine and to the middle of the septum, and the anterior palatine goes to the lower and middle turbinates. The olfactory nerve enters the nose through twelve openings of the oribriform plate – distributed to the special nerves adjacent to the mucous membrane of the superior turbinate.

Dr Paul Gillet was awarded the Légion d'honneur by the French

Minister of Public Health. This was an exception to the usual rule as this great honour was normally only awarded to members of the Medical Corps who either occupied an official post in a hospital or who held a professorship in the Faculty of Medicine.

This doctor was a house physician in a hospital and was formerly head of the Laboratory of the Faculty of Medicine, but had no official standing. He did most of his research in the privacy of his own home. He worked independently and was thus able to make more progress than most of his colleagues occupying administrative posts.

You may wonder what Dr Paul Gillet discovered which, at the time, aroused so much public attention. In 1929 he defined and fixed certain principles of use for his methods. He was scoffed at by his fellow doctors only because they had not understood his methods and had applied them incorrectly. Dr Gillet threw fresh light upon his work, he increased its possibilities and thus was born what was then known as 'Sympathico Therapy' (the therapy of stimulating the sympathetic nervous system by exciting the nasal passages with nasal probes or stylets).

He was the first man to prove that by massaging the mucous membrane of the nasal passage by means of metal stylets, communication could be established with that part of the nervous system called the sympathetic system. He went to great lengths to demonstrate that the sympathetic nervous system, a particularly mysterious set of nerves, was present in the midst of the nasal mucous membrane in the form of countless thousands of terminal strands grouped in a mass.

Once this premise is understood, it is very easy to conceive how the slightest disturbance arising in the midst of this vast intricate plexus is liable to have infinite repercussions, sometimes affecting the whole organism.

As a matter of fact if, instead of being constituted haphazardly, the science of medicine were still to be founded on scientific grounds, its creators would undoubtedly be saying, 'Above all, let us focus our attention on the sympathetic system. Let us watch over its functional activities, fathom its secrets, and study its immense possibilities.' The sympathetic nervous system controls the flow of blood – it is thus the master of life and death, well-being and suffering, illness and health.

Devote yourself to a thorough study of the sympathetic nervous system as did Dr Paul Gillet. It was he who brought to light the fact that when the mucous membrane of the nose is touched, the sympathetic system is awakened.

It has also been demonstrated that the effect of the communication thus established in the sympathetic system was to awaken it, and also restore its balance, with the result that apparent miracles and rapid cures were effected in many serious and previously 'incurable' diseases.

The nervous system, as we understand it, consists of two parts. One is situated in the brain and bone marrow, and on this depend our will and motor power – our will, thought, action, power, effort, ability to see and hear, all depend on the cerebro-spinal system.

Besides these important functions, there exists others which are obscure, involuntary and automatic; the beating of the heart, the blood circulation, the digestion of the stomach and intestines, the secretion of internal glands – the balance and well-being of our organism depend on the sympathetic nervous system.

The domain is therefore primordial. It might perhaps be conceived that an organism could exist without a cerebro-spinal system by leading a form of vegetable life. But without a sympathetic nervous system it would be impossible to exist. Just consider for a moment . . . without the sympathetic nervous system the blood would immediately cease to circulate and thus the cerebro-spinal system could no longer fulfil its functions.

The sympathetic nervous system consists of a series of nerve ganglions situated about one inch on either side of the spinal vertebrae (column). From these ganglions branch millions of strands surrounding each of the cells of which our body is made up: the cells of the muscles, bones, cartilage, viscera and even of the brain.

It was once stated by the founder of osteopathy, Dr Andrew Still, that the artery reigns supreme. This means that the blood flow must be unimpeded to maintain life itself. The sympathetic plexus exercises absolute control over each cell in the body, by regulating the flow of blood, which is the bearer of the oxygen and food, and also the transmitter of cellular secretion.

With this idea in mind, sympathetic therapy was created. It involves massaging the mucous membrane of the nose and mouth for a few seconds. It is an established fact that the brain and marrow float in a layer of fluid (the cephalorachidian liquid). The pressure of the fluid is greatly increased as soon as the mucous membrane of the nose is touched or irritated. At the same time, the number of leucocytes in the blood is profoundly modified. These alterations prove unquestionably that the application of the nasal technique is not just a superficial formality.

Yoga's rhythmic breathing is Nature's way of energising the membranes. The longer the breath, the longer the irritation and the more powerful the sympathetic reflex. Nature has it that only one nostril flows in each hour, except momentarily during changeover, when both nostrils flow. This is Nature's way of not over-exciting the nasal reflex.

Each nostril has its time and rhythm of flow. Thus when the left nostril is flowing, one is taking in and exciting the negative side of the body. Alternatively, when the right nostril is flowing, one is taking in and exciting the positive side of the body. During the 'changeover' a neutralising breath is taken when both nostrils flow. This is the neutral side of the energy or the blending of these energies. Thus, you will observe that the body is maintained by this negative, positive and neutral flow of the life-giving energy in the breath we breathe. Orientals call it *Prana*, and Occidentals refer to it as *Nous*, which means 'the unknown but important quality'.

It should be noted that deep or rhythmic breathing stimulates and accelerates the nerve endings of the positive end of the body.

Always breathe through the nose, as breathing through the mouth will not only endanger our sense of smell, but our mouth will dry up and infection can easily develop. Walking in the fresh air, a healthy diet and physical exercise – swimming, walking, cycling – will all be beneficial. If necessary, boost the body's immunity with Imuno-Strength from Nature's Best. Alternatively, take a glass of hot water with the juice of half a lemon and thirty drops of Echinaforce to reinforce resistance. In cases of breathing difficulties, use the Lymph Drops from Enzymatic Therapy.

THE THROAT AND RESPIRATORY SYSTEM

I have seen many sore throats that have been neglected. Doctors used to look at the tongue, which can tell us many stories about what goes on inside the body. Indeed, the tongue is an excellent diagnostic tool. The Chinese, however, believe that we should look at a patient's throat, as throats can become hotbeds of bacteria. This is indeed true, and prevention of a sore throat is very important. For this purpose Dr Vogel has always recommended Molkosan, the whey of the milk. Molkosan has an antiseptic quality, and is of great benefit as a throat gargle or when swallowed. It is also recommended for the treatment of diabetes. Sore throats and laryngitis can often result when the immune system is overstressed. In today's society we are increasingly susceptible to throat ailments and, without doubt, we have a great build-up of mucus because of pollution. The figures for asthma and bronchitis have escalated as a result of pollution.

For any problems with the respiratory tract, diet is very important. Limit the intake of dairy foods and salt. The mucous membranes are the organs which help to eliminate toxins. When we indulge in the wrong foods such as dairy produce, starchy foods, pasta and chocolate, the mucous membranes will react. When laryngitis and pharyngitis develop, gargling with a small amount of Molkosan and taking a little extra Echinaforce daily we can keep this under control.

With rhinitis and sinusitis also limit the intake of dairy foods and salt, but honey is advised. Take the homoeopathic Formula SNS twice a day (ten drops before meals), Lymph Drops after meals and take some Imuno-Strength twice a day.

Our immune system is a multi-faceted, highly sophisticated system which helps to protect our bodies and keep them healthy. The maintenance of an efficient immune system is dependent upon adequate intakes of certain vitamins and minerals that are included in Imuno-Strength. Vitamins, minerals and amino acids are essential to health and vitality. Although these substances occur naturally in various foods, adequate nutrition is not always achieved. Often, even in a well-planned diet, the vitamin and mineral status may be reduced or destroyed by poor cooking and preparation methods. People with inadequate diets, immune dysfunction, chronic illness, periods of rapid growth, behavioural disturbances and delinquencies, the institutionalised and the elderly may all be at risk from dietary deficiencies.

The formation of components of the immune system places an increased demand on the body, as do other physical or mental challenges. People who may benefit from this remedy include those who are recovering from illness, surgery and trauma.

When I was a child in the Netherlands it was the trend for children to have the tonsils removed at the first sign of infection. My mother was very much against this, but we had no option. Unfortunately, my tonsils became inflamed and the decision was made to remove them. I have always regretted this decision, because the tonsils protect the throat. When there is a definite need for their removal and it has to be done, then of course there is no choice. In severe and chronic cases of tonsillitis or if they are enlarged, a tonsillectomy may be necessary. Alternatively, I have found that the homoeopathic remedy *Lachesis* is capable of shrinking swollen tonsils, and gargling with Molkosan is also helpful. To combat infection, the American remedy Phyto-Biotic is beneficial and often replaces an antibiotic. Echinaforce will also be of help.

In cases of an abscess or interference with the larynx develops, immediate action must be taken. I have met too many people who have neglected this or delayed seeking treatment and their voice has become affected.

When the respiratory system is under attack the supply of oxygen through the lungs and into the bloodstream is restricted. The lungs are two elastic spongy organs that will serve us well, if only we take care of them. Normal breathing frequency in an adult should be 11 to 16 times per minute.

The following plants are very helpful for the respiratory system: Icelandic moss, eucalyptus, galeopsis, hedera helix, hyssop, inula, peppermint, pine, pimpinella. Two remedies formulated by Dr Vogel are also useful: Bronchosan, which is a combination remedy for congestion, and Santasapina, a pine needle cough syrup (to be taken one teaspoon twice a day in a cup of hot water).

During the winter, when viruses and colds abound, a vitamin C supplement is recommended. Vitamin C with bioflavonoids from Nature's Best is especially good for acute colds. This is a hypoallergenic formulation of vitamin C, rosehip and bioflavonoids. Vitamin C and bioflavonoids occur together in Nature. One of the richest sources of this combination is found in the pulp and rind of citrus fruits and certain vegetables. Bioflavonoids occur naturally as organic plant pigments that appear to assist in the absorption of vitamin C, and they are particularly important for maintaining the integrity of the blood vessels as they support collagen manufacture. Some bioflavonoids have anti-oxidant properties rather like vitamin C, and have been shown to protect both vitamin C and adrenalin from oxidation by copper-containing enzymes. Rosehip syrup in its undiluted form is one of the richest sources of vitamin C, and was used to promote health long before vitamin C was discovered. This combination of vitamin C, rosehip powder and bioflavonoids provides those who have dietary insufficiency with adequate vitamin C to supplement their diets.

When suffering from a cold, a blocked nose can be cleared by placing a thinly sliced onion by the bed. A hot bath with a few drops of an essential oil such as eucalyptus or Po-Ho oil from Bioforce, can also be helpful. To relieve stubborn conditions take Aconite D4 (three times a day, ten drops) or Pulsatilla D6 (every two hours, ten drops). Urticalcin (take twice a day, five tablets before meals) is a homoeopathic calcium, mixed with nettle extract, which is easily absorbed by the bloodstream.

It is often said that a common cold is best left alone, but I do not agree with this, as it can easily develop into asthmatic or bronchitic problems. It is estimated that in Britain two hundred million colds occur annually, leading to the loss of nearly four million working days. The rhino virus is the most likely culprit and causes a stuffed-up nose, headaches and blocked sinuses.

If there is susceptibility to common colds, as well as taking the remedies I have suggested, zinc can be helpful. Nature's Best produces Zinc Plus Lozenges, which should be sucked slowly for maximum effect. The principal role of any trace element is that of promoting the catalytic action of enzymes. Zinc is an invaluable mineral, which plays a role in the dehydrogenation and peptidase processes. It is specific for carboxypeptidase, which is the enzyme that removes the terminal amino acid from the carboxy end of a peptide. It is also specific for carboxylic anhydrase, the enzyme responsible for the ultimate elimination of carbon dioxide from an organism, and in the production of hydrochloric acid in the parietal cells of the stomach mucosa. Zinc is also an integral part of insulin, the hormone used for the treatment of diabetes, and is essential for all protein synthesis in the body. Any extra physical or mental demands made on the body can increase the need for zinc or cause our bodies to lose extra zinc, whereas phytate and fibre-rich foods inhibit the absorption of zinc from food.

One fifth of zinc in the body is found in the skin. Zinc helps tissue renewal and is involved in some of the enzymatic reactions necessary for the skin's normal oil gland function. The health of several body systems such as the nervous, immune and reproductive systems are influenced by zinc, as are the senses of taste and smell.

Hot steam infusions of essential oils, such as peppermint, eucalyptus and thyme will have a soothing effect on respiratory conditions. It is also a great help to use some extra enzymes because an enzyme deficiency can inhibit the absorption of essential vitamins and minerals.

Diet is also very important. The diet should contain extra proteins, plenty of fruit and vegetable juices, lemon, orange, garlic and some olive oil. Salt should be kept to a minimum. For problems with asthma and bronchitis, garlic, onions, honey, vegetables, protein-rich foods and propolis should feature in the diet, whereas dairy produce should be avoided.

Case histories

I remember a 75-year-old patient who had suffered from asthma for many years and latterly had lost his senses of smell and taste. He also complained of arthritis. I noticed that the air passages to the lungs were very inflamed; probably during his working life he had been subjected to a dusty atmosphere. Moreover, he was also a smoker. He brought some notes with him from the hospital with the results of recent tests. For his arthritis I prescribed

Imperthritica (twice a day, 15 drops) and also GS-Complex (twice a day, one capsule). For the asthma I gave him four tablets of Kelpasan, to be taken in the morning. I also prescribed ASM drops from Bioforce and three garlic capsules to be taken at night. I advised him against milk and cheese and suggested he drink plenty of fruit juices. Within a short time he was able to reduce his respiratory drugs and inhalers and his condition improved. He realised that he was getting better when he was once again able to appreciate the smell of coffee.

A world-famous singer consulted me because she had lost her sense of taste and smell. Worse still, she also felt that her voice had changed, and not for the better. When I made my diagnosis by looking, listening and feeling, I noticed that one of her jaw bones was slightly out of place. I was very sorry for her because I know that she is so talented. With the help of manipulative treatment I released the TM (temporo-mandibular) joint, which took the pressure off the hyoid bone. This gave her immediate relief. I then told her that she should drink plenty of enzyme-rich juices, e.g. bilberry, beetroot and artichoke. I prescribed Emergency Essence and Vitality Essence, and told her to use aromatherapy oils with steam baths. Together with manipulation of the joint, these resolved her problem and it was unbelievable that after three weeks her senses of taste and smell returned.

A 37-year-old female patient complained of feeling constantly exhausted and depressed. She had recently visited her dentist to have dentures fitted and after this had lost her senses of taste and smell. When I examined her tongue I could see it was coated and her throat was slightly inflamed. One of the main reasons for her problems was that the artificial dentures had a detrimental influence on her saliva. Because she was so depressed I gave her Jay Vee, which is a herbal combination that I formulated some years ago. This remedy contains a blend of natural substances including valerian (*Valeriana officinalis*), *Crataegus* (hawthorn) and *Humulus lupulus* (hop), which gained popularity in the nineteenth century. Passiflora, a plant often admired for its beautiful colours, is also present, and zinc for its function connected with the immune system. I further suggested that she should use sage for her physical tiredness, and to promote energy she should use the essential oils rosemary, basil and marjoram in the bath. I also advised her to see an aromatherapist.

Finally, I recommended that she take Co-Enzyme Q10 (twice a day, 10 mg). Co-Enzyme Q10 or Ubiquinone, which means 'everywhere', is a normal and essential component of the mitochondria. The mitochondria are the energy generators of the cells and the highest proportion of these are found in the cells that do the most work, notably in the liver, muscle tissue and the heart. This co-enzyme is essential for the health of all human tissues and organs. It is a vitamin-like substance which is made in the body and can be found in some foods, but seems difficult to extract from them. A food supplement of CoQ10 may be useful to help ensure that there is an ample level of this important co-factor in the tissues at all times. CoQ10 was first discovered in humans by Dr Leonard Mervyn, and researchers are still uncovering the full extent of CoQ10's role in our metabolism.

Leading scientists believe that CoQ10 is, in effect, a 'biochemical spark' or catalyst that releases energy from food. It is therefore involved when we exert physical energy. Studies in the USA and Belgium have shown that obese people have lower levels of CoQ10 in their tissue cells than those who are slim, as do people taking cholesterol-lowering medication.

This combination of remedies helped this patient so that she soon returned to normal.

I shall never forget the gentleman in his forties who came to see me with a neck problem. He told me that he had been stretching at work when suddenly he had felt a sharp pain in his neck. He was almost doubled up in pain but at that time he omitted to tell me that he had also lost the senses of smell and taste. The most common problems in the neck usually involve the third or fourth cervical vertebra. I noticed after rotation and examination that in this case it was the first cervical vertebra. This is not the easiest manipulation for an osteopath, but I adapted an old-fashioned method and adjusted the ears and worked the tongue. I could see the relief on his face. After three days he returned, overjoyed because his senses of smell and taste had come back after being absent for several years.

3

Taste

'I would give anything in the world to regain my sense of taste,' confided a pleasant grey-haired gentleman to me. 'Not only have I lost my sense of smell, but my sense of taste has also gone. Food used to be one of my passions, but now I no longer enjoy smell or taste. I know that I never really appreciated these senses until I have had to do without.'

When people lose their senses of taste and smell they are devastated, as it is true that we rarely appreciate these pleasures until we have to do without them. Although our palate can become used to many things, when our senses of taste or smell become affected, we lose what may be considered some of the primary pleasures in life. It is also a lesson for people with a weight problem that the palate may be re-educated to like wholesome foods, such as fresh fruits and vegetables, instead of packaged and processed foods with artificial flavours. Such foods are not only lacking in nutritional value, but they also do nothing to stimulate our tastebuds.

Taste is a very valuable commodity and one of the reasons I am writing about this subject is that all too often I hear people complain that they regret their loss of the sense of taste, or indeed any one or more of the five senses. Today's society is threatened by pollution and interference in the three forms of energy we live by, i.e. food, water and air, and this should not be regarded lightly.

If we think of taste, it is most likely that we first of all associate this with our tongue. Some time ago I awoke in the night in a lot of pain, which I soon discovered was caused by an infected tooth. Because the pain was so penetrating I decided to use some oil of cloves, which indeed helped to dull the pain. However, for several days I lost all sense of taste and also experienced a numbness of the tongue. That taught me that people who often eat highly spiced foods, with such a power of penetration, can find their tastebuds are numbed for long periods at a time. If such meals are an exception, our tastebuds will recover, but if we regularly overdose on strong spices in our diet, the tastebuds will eventually lose their full sensitivity. I had good reason to be grateful that Nature is so resilient, because in my case I regained my sense of taste within a few days.

There are many conditions that can be responsible for affecting our sense of taste, and sometimes smell. The tongue may sometimes be coated with lesions, which reduce our sense of taste, or it may be caused by stomatitis, which is an oral inflammation. It could also be due to conditions such as the fairly common *Herpes simplex*, or an ailment called glossitis. The latter is an acute chronic inflammation of the tongue. In fact, there are numerous causes that can temporarily, or permanently, affect our ability to enjoy taste. However, in the *Merck Manual* we read that since disorders of smell or taste are not life-threatening, they often fail to receive close medical attention. Nevertheless, they can be a great loss, and also a detrimental influence on our other senses.

When we study the tongue we can hardly fail to be surprised at the cleverness of Creation, even if we only think of it as an indicator of our well-being, because the tongue is like a chart of our general health. The nerve cells that register the sensation of taste and transmit it to the brain number in excess of 3,000. To think that we have this fantastic mechanism and that the different taste zones of the tongue are accurate and reliable and experienced tasters! They are like a well-tuned chemical laboratory. What would life be like without these 3,000 tastebuds? And isn't it strange to realise that this relatively small part of man's anatomy has such a far-reaching function?

I have heard Dr Vogel observe in some of his lectures that horses and ships are more easily managed than the tongue. The tongue not only provides us with our sense of taste, it also gives us the power of speech or silence. Just think how profound is the saying: 'to hold one's tongue'.

In her excellent book *The Natural History of our Senses*, Diane Ackerman writes about taste in a social sense. She states that our first sense of taste is the milk from our mother's breast. That is provided with feelings of love and affection, with stroking, and a sense of security and warmth. She stresses that the quality of what we eat and drink is very important. Our tastebuds are exceedingly small and not only are they found on the tongue, but also on the palate, the tonsils and the pharynx.

It should always be remembered that the foodstuffs we usually crave tend to be the worst foods for us. We see that with alcoholics, as well as with chocaholics. Yet it is not beyond our ability to retrain our senses, and this often requires no more than a healthy dose of willpower combined with a general understanding of what is happening in our body.

The endocrine system plays a large role in all the five senses and if there is a loss of any of these senses, this is sometimes overcome involuntarily when I prescribe a course of treatment for the endocrine or immune system. The tongue needs exercise – that means more than just speaking, as it concerns the *way* we use our voice. The energies of the five senses should be in harmony. It may sound extreme, but it is a fact that even minor vibrations play a role here. If we lose our sense of touch, smell, taste, hearing or vision we should appreciate that this is usually the result of a disharmony somewhere in the body. If we understand why this loss has occurred, we can find ways to correct the situation.

Every molecule and every atom of the universe – animate and inanimate – is in constant vibration. Each mineral and each life cell in man, animal, or insect, vibrates on its own frequency and wavelength. Also, there are vibrations of sound, colour and smell, of heat and light. In addition, the earth and all its living things are continuously being bombarded by stellar vibrations and cosmic rays of a frequency too high for us to comprehend. Furthermore, the earth is surrounded and criss-crossed by magnetic bands, man-made radio currents, all vibratory in nature. These are facts and governed by the laws of Nature.

Vibrations of sound can cause pleasure or pain according to their effect on our emotions. A rhythmic tune will start our feet tapping involuntarily, while a plaintive melody will often bring a lump to the throat and cause tears. A dog will cry out in pain at the blast of a whistle and will howl painfully at the strains of a violin. There is also power in the human voice – power to influence or to offend. The ancient peoples knew the power of the spoken word, which is borne out by the old proverb: 'A soft answer turneth away wrath.'

Most powerful of all, yet the least understood, are the cosmic vibrations. There can be no doubt that they exercise a profound influence on our lives.

Cosmic vibrations are open to all of us, but it all depends if we are open to them. It has been said that the pineal gland is the cosmic aerial. We can easily influence it by spending our days staring at a computer monitor or a word processor, or spending hours inactively gazing at a television screen. The endocrine glands, of which the pineal gland is one, should be in tune with Nature, and with our Creation. In other words, we must endeavour to ease our communication with Nature. We often come across this when people talk about our 'sixth sense', an expression that seems to refer to something mysterious. Basically, it means that what in humans is called intuition, and in animals instinct, makes us unusually sensitive and perceptive to intangible changes and influences.

THE ENDOCRINE AND OTHER KEY GLANDS – THEIR FUNCTION AND MALFUNCTION

The endocrine system is made up of seven proportionally small glands, yet these seven glands are of great influence on our five tangible senses. You will know that I maintain that there are seven colours in the rainbow, seven light receptors in the retina of the eye, seven layers of light, and seven basic steps in a musical octave. Harmony is of the essence. Looking at colours we discover the beauty of Nature, as well as the power of colour therapy, but I will come back to that in the chapter on vision. However, I want to emphasise here how remarkably effective colour therapy is in the treatment of the endocrine system. If there is no harmony in the endocrine system, there is great danger that one or more of the senses will suffer.

The elementary principles of colour therapy are as follows:

- The pineal gland reacts to violet.
- The pituitary gland reacts to indigo.
- The thymus gland reacts to green.
- The thyroid gland reacts to blue.
- The pancreas reacts to yellow.
- The adrenals react to orange.
- The gonad glands react to red.

Our bodies may be compared to a car. There are two conditions for its efficient operation: the machinery must be in good working order, and it must be supplied with suitable fuel. Taking this point a little further, in the body, the endocrines function in a similar way to the carburettors and the autonomic system to the tuning and wiring systems.

It is a sorry fact that very little is known or recorded on the subject of endocrine function or malfunction. The endocrines are the lifeline of the human system and if they could be fully understood and the resulting knowledge applied, the ability to alleviate many symptoms of ill health would be in our grasp.

There are methods of influencing the endocrines (physical methods) by use and control through areas of the feet, and also vital areas in the cranial vault. It has long been a misconception that the chakras control the endocrines – nothing could be further from the truth. The chakras are the whirling vortices that circulate the polarity energy to all parts of the human body. In so doing, these vortices nourish the energies of the endocrine system, but these chakras are *not* the endocrine system.

A few things to note and remember:
- The result of motion is the production of energy.
- If a gland has energy and vibration, it is active.
- Every gland serves as a specific workshop or laboratory for the preparation of certain substances. These enter the bloodstream and are utilised to maintain the integrity of the body.
- These glands represent *balance in the body*.
- The parotid gland controls the endocrines.
- The physical activity of a person is greatly dependent upon his body chemistry. This is controlled and regulated by his ductless or endocrine glands.

The endocrine system exists for the purpose of maintaining the correct state of blood protein and tissue colloids.

- The emotions activate the adrenals.
- The adrenals act on the nervous system.
- The nervous system affects the sympathetics.
- The adrenals link into the thyroid and parasympathetics.

The mechanism control for the healthy functioning of the body consists of the pituitary-hypothalamus complex: the pituitary supervises and influences the glandular system; the hypothalamus supervises and influences the autonomic system. The hypothalamus is *sensory*.

The brain holds in the thalamus, a fluid which gives balance to the head, like a spirit level. It is a form of blood plasma and flows over the nervous system. In the pineal gland and the thalamus all things are comprehended.

THE PINEAL GLAND
The main function of this gland is control over the development of the sex apparatus and body growth (generative, skeletal and somatic). It also supports the sensory and motor nerves to the eyes.

The pineal and thymus glands work in harmony. If overactive in puberty, serious results follow.

The pineal gland, or aerial to the body, is very attuned to cosmic influences and needs relaxation and meditation. In cases of cancer consider carefully the state of the pineal and thymus glands. The pathology usually shows in the formation of cysts and tumours. Even hydrocephalus may develop, due to pressure on the veins of galen and the aquaduct of sylvius.

Signs and symptoms of imbalance

1. Early growth, often premature as well as mental and sexual precocity in children
2. Decreased sexual power in adults
3. Polymuria, adiposity and later defectiveness
4. Neuralgia and pressure signs
5. Precocious mental, genital and somatic development
6. Tumours of various types
7. Tumour causing pyloric obstruction and vagus interference, resulting in epilepsy

THE PITUITARY GLAND

The *anterior pituitary* maintains mental equilibrium and activates the brain cells. It is responsible for brain capacity and mental control. It promotes growth in all bones and tissue, and promotes lactation.

The anterior pituitary produces several endocrines, which are as follows:

1. Growth endocrines
2. Sex-stimulating endocrines
3. Thyrotrophic endocrines
4. Adrenotrophic endocrines: to medulla – to cortex
5. Diabetogenic endocrines
6. Pancreatic endocrines

If it is out of balance we would have an unstable mentality, lack of control and unbalanced sex organs. Consider the possibility of diabetes if the anterior pituitary is low as it promotes production of insulin.

The *posterior pituitary* is composed of nervous tissue. It stimulates the nervous system and regulates the water metabolism, stimulates contraction of the muscles in the body, influences metabolism and increases the respiration. It secretes pitressin, which produces the following effects:

1. Raises the blood pressure
2. Is diuretic and anti-diuretic
3. Influences obesity through water retention
4. Increases stomach and intestinal secretions
5. Is antagonistic to insulin

The secretion pitressin is a vaso constrictor. It is closely related to the suprarenals, the gonads, the thyroid and the thymus.

The posterior pituitary is a thermal centre and burns up water, carbohydrates and fat. It is responsible for metorraghia and menorraghia. Worry has an effect on the posterior pituitary.

Normalising the glands, in general, brings about new hair growth. Cases of haemorrhage can be stopped by normalising the parathyroids. The treatment of the parathyroids relieves asthma. In abortion, consider the anterior pituitary and the ovaries. In deafness, consider the pituitary, the thyroid and the ovaries. In dementia look at the pituitary and the thyroid. In diabetes insipidus look to the posterior pituitary. In eczema look to the pituitary, the thyroid and the pancreas.

THE THYROID

The main functions of the thyroid are as follows:

1. Secretes thyroxin – it is released when iodine is low in the circulation
2. Controls or regulates the metabolism
3. Sensitises every cell and organ of the body to sympathetic stimulation
4. Assists in control of tissue differentiation
5. Increases the heart rate
6. Controls coagulation
7. Increases urea and fluid secretion

8. Stimulates mental alertness
9. Controls and regulates fat
10. Controls intestinal motility

Its relationship with the other endocrines is as follows:

1. It is antagonistic to insulin in the pancreas.
2. The thyroid and the medulla of the suprarenals are synergetic.
3. A close relationship exists between the thyroid and the gonads.
4. It is antagonistic to the parathyroids.
5. It acts on and is acted on by the pituitary – these being known as the thyrotropic and the adrenotropic, etc.

In cases of thyroid hyperfunction, the individual is quick, vivacious, and mentally and physically alert. Symptoms might include tachycardia and exophthalmus. Extreme cases may lead to Grave's disease. Hypothyroid would present a sluggish mentality, generalised obesity, fat above the clavicle and back of hands, slow pulse, low blood pressure and a continual feeling of coldness. The thyroid has a specific action upon brain cells and the sympathetic nervous system. If wounds heal slowly, look at the thyroid. The thyroid directly influences all the other endocrine glands. Not only does the kidney function decrease with hyperthyroid trouble but also the arteries, the heart action, while the sensory and motor nerves increase in function.

THE PARATHYROIDS

While they are not strictly endocrine glands themselves, the parathyroids are definitely under the control of the two energies of the body, i.e. the left by the energy in the blood and the right by nervous energy. They will slow down the action of the sex glands in a normal person. Any person needs the parathyroids above all other glands. Moreover, the parathyroids will stimulate all the endocrines. Other functions are as follows:

1. Regulate calcium in the blood and tissue
2. Increase intestinal peristalsis

3. Regulate absorption and excretion of mineral salts in the body
4. Maintain the neuro-muscular balance and sympathetic equilibrium
5. Detoxicate
6. Necessary in coagulation of milk and blood
7. With trypsinogen, they assist protein metabolism
8. Through calcium balance, they regulate the heart rhythm
9. Through calcium balance, they regulate the permeability of the cell membranes and thereby assist in controlling allergic conditions

The upper-right parathyroid controls toxins, calcium and the function of the nerves of the head and neck. The lower-right parathyroid controls toxins, calcium and the functions of the nerves of the body and limbs.

The glands regulate the distribution of calcium in the body, build fat, control muscle and nerve irritability, and aid in detoxication. They also stimulate the suprarenals to secrete adrenalin. The parathyroids are governed by the pituitary; they sustain the mammary glands and pancreas, as both these use carbon.

Tetany is usually due to the inefficient function of the parathyroids. Calcium control is lacking, allowing the neuro-muscular impulse to go uninterrupted. Hyperfunction of the parathyroids will lead to decalcification of the bone, where they begin to resemble soap bubbles in appearance. Usually there is a tumour in one or more of the glands. It causes calcium to be mobilised from the bone and makes bones brittle. The bones sometimes even become soft.

It is advisable to normalise the parathyroids in cases of haemorrhage as this assists the calcium mobilisation. The calcium converts prothrombin into thrombin and helps clotting.

Calcium united with phosphorus to form calcium phosphate, which is needed in low-grade cases, i.e. cancer, tuberculosis and pernicious anaemia.

Hyperfunction of the parathyroids results from low calcium reproduction. It soothes the nerves and muscles, and controls the speed at which the impulses are carried into the neuro-muscular system. Usually there is a complete lack of tone in all muscles, also in the intestines, and slow digestion and elimination of pancreatic juices and gastric juices.

THE THYMUS
The thymus influences growth and is thought to be connected with the lymphocytes. This gland is made up of lymphoid tissues. Infection diseases seem to cause the thymus to atrophy.

The two great controlling glands are the thymus (in the case of the mind) and the parathyroid (in the case of the emotions and physical aspects). In some cases of asthma, the thymus function is found to be deficient. When this gland is operating inefficiently, creative mental power decreases. I am convinced that the thymus and parathyroids are glands which reduce levels of activity and act as controls.

Always think of the thymus gland where there is not only sensitivity to physical stimuli, but to mental ones as well.

THE SPLEEN
The chief function of the spleen is that of a detoxicant – and it is always involved in a toxic condition. It removes dead cells. Hyperfunction can cause extreme anaemia. The spleen is usually involved in typhoid, typhus, malaria and severe forms of anaemia. The lymph and suprarenals are always associated with the spleen.

This gland is high in sulphur. The spleen is responsible for maintaining the composition of the circulatory blood at certain levels. If the gland is not well balanced, the brain will not function properly. A patient has a better fighting chance if the spleen is in good condition.

The spleen is liable to be depleted in typhoid, malaria or other low-grade fevers. In cases of anaemia, an increased intake of sulphuric-rich foods is advised. Garlic has a very high sulphur content. The spleen and liver are closely allied. Dysfunction can cause hyperacidity, acidosis or general toxaemia. When the spleen becomes inactive, the lymph nodes and bone may attempt to carry on its function.

In acute spleen conditions the spleen becomes soft and flabby. In chronic spleen conditions the spleen is felt to be hard.

Important symptoms which indicate a possible spleen condition are enlargement, tenderness on pressure, and a feeling of weight. If there is high blood pressure with enlargement, there may be a very discernible pulsation over the spleen.

This organ assists in the control of water storage and circulation. If constant fear and worries persist, it will draw the entire endocrine wheel out of balance. If the individual experiences an emotion such as fear or terror, resulting in an outpouring of adrenalin, and if the cortex is added, it turns to anger.

THE PANCREAS

The pancreas concerns itself with the digestive tract. It is a gland of digestion. Its main function is the secretion of insulin, which maintains the blood sugar at the normal level. In addition, it aids in the metabolism of fats and in the absorption of carbohydrates, e.g. glucose. It also converts glycogen back to glucose when needed.

The pancreas is closely related to the liver, suprarenals and the pituitary. The liver and suprarenals are regulated by the pituitary. If the head of the pancreas is low in function, the patient will be unable to cope with starch. If the tail of the pancreas is low in function, the patient cannot take sweets, has mouth canker and swollen gums. If the Islets of Langerhans are low in function, the patient will crave sugar but cannot take it. Consider the possibility of *Diabetes mellitus. Diabetes mellitus* is a condition that can affect any age, but it is to be suspected in a patient over fifty years if he becomes erratic or irritable, and experiences weakness, insomnia or intense craving.

Diabetes may be accompanied by all manner of digestive disturbances, skin irritation, carbuncles, cataract, neuritis, acidosis, etc. There are many other conditions showing excess sugar, e.g. pneumonia, typhoid, cancer or tuberculosis, but each has its various diagnostic points.

The pancreas gives its support to the skin and kidneys. It should be considered in both the diagnosis and treatment of epilepsy (usually the tail of the pancreas is involved), together with the pineal in cases of epileptic seizures. In hypertension, look for imbalance in the tail of the pancreas, also the thyroid, the ovaries and the suprarenals. In all infections and cases of low blood pressure look at the tail of the pancreas. The same area is relevant for gastric ulcers, skin ulcers and irritation of the skin.

THE SUPRARENALS

These furnish tone and strength to every tissue and organ in the body. They select calcium for the bloodstream. The medulla secretes adrenalin and the cortex produces an external secretion known as cortin.

The main functions of the medulla are as follows:

1. Increases heartbeat and blood pressure
2. Contracts the uterus and all mucous membranes through the sympathetic system
3. Helps to reduce peristalsis
4. Stimulates kidney function and metabolism
5. Contrary to other gland action, it dilates the pupils
6. Decreases coagulation time – contracts the blood vessels
7. Stimulates smooth muscles

In the case of the cortex, the main functions are as follows:

1. Assists in control of renal function and extraction of sodium
2. Assists in carbohydrate metabolism
3. Is important in body strength
4. Assists in sexual development
5. Opposes thyroxin
6. Stores vitamin C
7. May assist in lactation
8. May assist in detoxication
9. Controls hot flushes during the menopause

This gland is closely associated with the gonads, the thyroid, the spleen and the pituitary.

Hypofunction of the medulla is indicated by general lack of tone and muscular weakness, e.g. influenza, forms of anaemia, chronic rheumatism, sinus problems, chronic prostitis, intestinal toxaemia, malignancies.

With hypofunction of the cortex, if the patient is over fifty years of age, losing weight and has low blood pressure, you should consider the possibility of Addison's disease. There are three conditions to differentiate: hypoadrenia, Addison's disease and pernicious anaemia. In all three the suprarenals would be of low function.

Where hyperfunction of the suprarenals is indicated, remember to take account of the patient's circulation and innervation, so their function is accentuated. Check the blood pressure, pulse and heart. Common symptoms are nervous fatigue and nervous exhaustion – the patient awakes exhausted. Some other signs are nervous irritability, an irritable heart and gastro-irritability.

The suprarenals come into their own when normalising an irregular or overactive heart.

THE OVARIES AND UTERUS

The ovaries activate the thyroid, stimulate the anterior pituitary, develop the ova and corpus luteum. Also produced in the ovaries is an internal secretion which is responsible for growth and development. Other functions of this search are as follows:

1. At puberty, it controls the growth of the mammary glands, vagina and uterus.
2. It assists in maintaining and producing the physical and psychic secondary sex characteristics.
3. It helps in the maintenance and establishment of the menstrual cycle.
4. In pregnancy, it aids the relaxation of the pubis and with the aid of the anterior pituitary it helps in the secretion of milk.

Low function of the ovaries can produce amenorrhoea, menopause, thyroid obesity (back and thighs). Hypofunction may cause arthritis, epilepsy, cardiovascular and nervous disturbances (the ovaries and thyroid are related) and it sensitises every organ and tissue in the body through the sympathetic nervous system. Usually, the cardiovascular disturbances would stem from obesity and toxin absorption. Predisposing factors to cause hypofunction include: inherited or constitutional disturbances, tumour, trauma, cysts, climacteric conditions, lack of tone through vitamin deficiency or glandular deficiency. In over- or hyperfunction one would find menorraghia, enlargement of the uterus, ovarian cysts or polypus growth on the uterus. Hypertension, hyperthyroidism or anaemiam tuberculosis may then follow. The anterior pituitary is allied to the ovaries and increases connective tissue: this would cause a uterine fibroid.

The uterus has three functions:
1. Menstruation
2. Pregnancy
3. Secretion of a hormone for mineral balance, the lack of which often causes rheumatism

Vitamin A is important for a healthy uterus and ovaries, and lack of vitamin E can lead to sterility. Arthritis is a common complaint in women and is usually due to ovarian insufficiency (corpus luteum). Agitation and worry will cause an imbalance in the ovaries which may result in hypo- or hyperactivity. The ovaries contribute to the well-being of the skin, hair, teeth, eyes, and both the motor and sensory nerves.

The ovaries should be considered in the following conditions: abortion, arteriosclerosis, arthralgia in the knee, small articulations of the hands, bladder irritation, bronchitis, bronchial pneumonia, common colds, deafness, haemorrhages during the menopause or puberty, menstrual headaches, obesity, tonsillitis, and vomiting during pregnancy.

THE TESTES AND PROSTATE
These are the male gonads, corresponding to the female ovaries, and very closely associated with the pituitary, the thyroid and the suprarenals. Their main functions are:

1. Primarily the production of the sperm
2. An internal secretion, which helps the secondary sex characteristics develop

3. The development and maintenance of the prostate sperm, the accessory
   sex apparatus
4. Growth and distribution of hair on the head and body
5. Maintaining the muscles of the larynx and the skeleton
6. Some control over fat distribution

Orchic hormones are formed which produce courage, optimism and mental control through their power to control the anterior pituitary.

In cases of hypofunction the following signs and symptoms would be apparent:

1. Small genitals and underdeveloped secondary sex characteristics
2. Overgrowth of long bones
3. High-pitched voice, generally feminine
4. Dental abnormalities
5. Clumsiness – dull and weak-minded attitude

Where an adult is affected, any of the following might result:

1. Regression of sexual characteristics, to varying degrees
2. Atrophy of the prostate
3. Girdle obesity
4. Nervous and psychic symptoms
5. Low resistance to infection and tendency to dementia, cirrhosis of the
   liver, parathyroid and thyroid disorders.

Conversely, hyperfunction could be indicated by:

1. Precocious puberty
2. Excessive development of sex organs
3. Rapid skeletal growth, resulting in short arms and legs
4. Premature tooth eruptions, separation, malfunction and overcrowding
5. Nervous and mental symptoms; tachycardia and tremors

These glands supply the skin, the motor and sympathetic nerves. Where the following conditions occur we should pay particular attention to the gonads: arteriosclerosis, bladder irritation, bronchial pneumonia, pulmonary embolism, cardiac hypertrophy, myocardial insufficiency and sciatic conditions.

The gonadotrophic hormone is linked to and works with the vagus nerve and is parasympathetic. The thyrotrophic hormone is linked and works with the sympathetics. Hyperfunction of gonadotrophic makes people sleep well; the pulse is retarded and they usually complain of constipation and hyperacidity. Hyperfunction of thyrotrophic usually causes insomnia; the pulse is accelerated and peristalsis of the intestines is increased.

THE LINK BETWEEN OBESITY AND THE ENDOCRINES
Obesity arises through the metabolic process; food alone is not the cause. Obesity is an abnormal accumulation of fat in the subcutaneous or other tissues due to deficient oxidation of fats formed from starches.

The endocrines concerned are the pituitary, the gonads, the thyroid, the pancreas, and the suprarenal cortex. The entire pituitary may be at fault; the anterior lobe is concerned with the gonads. In pituitary obesity the fat is general, but especially deposited around the waist. The thyroid is the incinerator of the body. Persons with thyroid obesity sometimes look much larger than their actual weight. The anterior pituitary is usually at fault as it assists the water metabolism of the body.

In thyroid obesity, the fat is more or less evenly distributed over the body and the skin looks lifeless. It is usually accompanied by low blood pressure, erratic menstruation and a lazy and sluggish disposition. In cases of obesity the normalisation of the thyroid gland has produced almost phenomenal results.

MUSCLE CONTRACTION
A holistic approach is required in the treatment of any condition or illness. Sometimes there may be only minor indications, as was the case with a female patient of mine who suffered with muscle contractions. It is often overlooked that such spasmodic muscular contractions can have a negative influence on the five senses.

Muscle contractions are due to nerve impulses passing via a

123

spinal trunk nerve to the nerve endings of the muscle. In a normal healthy person such contraction, followed by relaxation, mainly during exercise, gives what is known as muscle tone. Such voluntary exercises improve the metabolism and increases the circulation of the blood which flows through the muscle; thus the muscle is permanently strengthened.

When the nerves, through disease or injury, are no longer able to conduct these nervous impulses, in the majority of cases muscle contraction is impossible.

When a muscle remains contracted, the result is fatigue, pain and other harmful effects. Its supply of oxygen is cut off and the blood and lymph being squeezed out of the tissues is affected.

When people talk glibly about tension what they have in mind is muscular tension. A muscle is capable of contraction and relaxation. Muscular spasm is another kettle of fish. The blood is squeezed out of a spastic muscle and oxygen cannot get to the tissues. Nature's warning is experienced as pain.

Everything in Nature is in a state of molecular tension. Otherwise, man, the moon, planets and other visible objects would disintegrate and fly off into space. Everything, then, is in motion. Nothing stands still. Stillness is death, destruction and change.

Tension is a natural function and state of being. It is the most important factor in physical life. It is responsible for the birth of a form, controlling the harmonious distribution of energy through its body. It is the *state of tension* that preserves the integrity of a form. The molecular construction of anything, be it animate or inanimate, is dependent upon this natural law of tension. Call it Life, Health or Cosmic Energy, it is the factor which prevents molecules from flying off into space. The tensile strength of a human cell is an electrical phenomena and is allied to its frequency or rate of vibration. When this is altered by faulty diet or even microbic invasion, the frequency and tension are also altered. The result is disease or disharmony.

Tension, as we know it, is muscular in nature, whether it be produced by the cold weather (we automatically tense ourselves) or other physical factor or emotional stimuli. We all know what happens when a muscle remains in a state of tension for any length of time, so I will not go into this.

Stress plays a significant role in this and if muscle contraction is combined with stress, much can be learned from the diagram in Figure 11, which was explained to me by a good friend of mine from the USA. It accounts for the glandular imbalance that results when stress rules our lives. Dr Hans Selye and other investigators have shown that some degree of stress in life is normal and may even be essential to healthy living. Most of us, however, are subjected to excessive stress in various forms. Stress frequency, intensity and duration largely determine the degree of altered body function, with resultant disorders and loss of resistance to disease. Thus excessive stress plays an important role in the disease process. Any disorder is a stress in itself and that is when the vicious circle begins.

To return again to tension, inner conflict, emotional upsets, etc. We are agreed that these factors, when they persist, actually precipitate soluble calcium from the bloodstream into the joints and bursae, and degenerative diseases such as arthritis, rheumatism and lumbago are likely to result.

The ability of the body to adequately cope with stress is

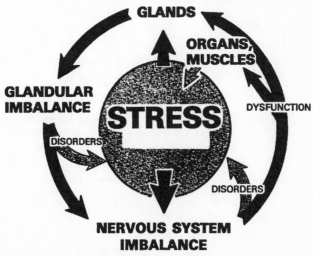

Figure 11: Stress Cycle

fundamental to good health. By correcting vertebral subluxation-fixations and balancing the body in other ways, the osteopath relieves major stresses on both the nervous system and the entire body. Osteopaths strive not only to relieve the effects or symptoms of dysfunction and disease, but to remove their causes, thus increasing the body's ability to restore and maintain optimum health.

The human frame is expertly formed, each muscle having its own inbuilt tension, its own inbuilt ability to contract or relax its fibres. Every member of the body is dependent on the muscles and life's processes could not continue to function without them.

Your physical condition is a good index of the state of your muscles. Vitality is indicative of good muscle tone and the opposite is also true when muscles lose their tonic quality and become flabby. You should have sufficient interest in your healing to want to understand the body muscles. It will repay you a thousand-fold. Study the controls through the nerve fibres that affect contraction and relaxation of the muscles.

Whatever the name given to disease, and there are more than a thousand such names, muscles are the basis of these aches and pains. A contracted muscle is a working muscle. It uses up nervous energy, consumes sugar and produces lactic acid – and this is the cause of ultimate fatigue.

To produce a state of relaxation in muscle tissue, apply pressure with the thumbs at both the origin and insertion of the muscle. This causes the muscle acids to be emptied and allows fresh nourishment to enter the fibres. The pressure should be maintained only for about ten to 20 seconds. In this way, normal muscle tone will soon be established, probably due to a vibration of the muscle itself produced by the cessation of fatigue.

The cellular and intercellular tensions must be corrected so as to remove all strain and thus bring all matter back to maximum usefulness by correction of fatigue.

Always check for muscle involvement in both pain and disease. Many years of research and experience has led us to understand the percentage of certain muscles and their involvement.

90% involvement	*80% involvement*
Anterior scalanus	Quadratas lumborum
Sub-scapularis	*70% involvement*
Sacro-spinalis	Tensor fascia lata
Pectoralis minor	*60% involvement*
Pectineus	Gracilis
Levitator angulae	Teres major
Infra-spinalus	Teres minor
Gluteus medius	*50% involvement*
Gluteus minimus	Adductor longus
Splenius capitis	*40% involvement*
Soleus	Piriformis
Gastrocnemius	

All other muscles become involved to a much lesser degree.

Stiffness of the muscles and ligaments will often have an influence on the inflammation of tissue. The stiffness is nearly always due to impeded venous circulation of the blood, or to the irritation of the nervous system, causing the muscular fibres to contract around nerve filaments and this increases the muscular contraction.

Disease is a condition of undue pressure (the interference of normal conditions, i.e. muscular contraction). It is an undisputable fact that when the nervous system is permitted to perform its normal function, disease cannot exist in the body.

The fact that all functions in the body are performed through the nervous system makes it imperative that we should fully understand the working of this system. When the nervous system is unduly interfered with, the result is disharmony. This is denoted by a diseased condition – as soon as harmony is restored, the disease ceases to exist. The aim should be 'take off the pressure': all will be free, Nature is satisfied, and friction ceases.

Muscular contraction is the cause of nerve pressure and the interference of nerve function. Relaxation becomes a necessity in order to permit the normal flow of fluids through the vessels.

It is a fact that disease is a result of violation of law, i.e. wrong thinking, either on the part of the individual or someone having control of the sick person. There can be no order anywhere unless the mind directs the forces, and this mind in man is the controlling power.

To know the condition is of more importance than the diagnosis, or the name of the disease. The nervous system controls every part of the human body and the functions of the five senses. Always remember that the nervous system is the medium through which all functions are performed. Inasmuch as normal tissue is a product of nerve influence and function, the mind, through the nerve filaments, has the entire supervision of the body in its power. It is logical to conclude that to relieve any abnormal condition, it is of prime importance to free the nervous system from all obstruction.

All rational human beings act as they think; hence all actions are the products of thought, excluding accidents and trauma. It is logical to assume that disease is also a product of thought. If disease were natural, then it would be wrong to use any means to relieve the person afflicted with disease.

Most methods of treatment, and this includes osteopathic treatments, do not adjust a subluxation or a lesion, but merely take off the pressure from the nervous system, which passes through the muscles along the spine.

RESTORING THE FLOW OF ENERGY

In China it is believed that the senses are the gates to all that happens. The senses are united with the universe. In effect, they are the windows of our whole being. These five senses remind us of the five wounds of Christ when he was nailed to the cross. Observation is the knowledge of truth. It should be understood when we study these five senses that are so closely linked with mind, body and soul, that medication and relaxation are essential for the development or improvement of senses.

Someone sent me a little book recently called *Who Am I?*, written by James Ashby and illustrated by a dear friend of mine, Alma Dowe. The words impressed me, but so did the illustrations. James Ashby wrote that in Hebrew the name of God is unpronounceable. Its letters are the base of 'To Be', and its sound is the sound of breathing. I read that our Creator gave us the breath of life, which influences our touch, our smell and our taste, affecting what we hear and what we see, and that we are a being, albeit minute, of the universe. In the early Christian Church Paul said that we are all sons and daughters of God. That is exactly what we are: part of that great Creation that I can meditate on with gratitude.

Whilst on this subject I am reminded of another book, for which I was invited to write the foreword: *Safe as Houses*. Written by David Curran and Rodney Girdleston, the book discloses many of the ways in which our health can be damaged. We read about the pros and cons of our dependency on modern technology. For example, David points out that the discovery of electricity is a wonder in itself, but we have taken it for granted. If we live under an electric field, which emits geopathic stress, are we aware that that same electricity could be harmful to our health? Electromagnetic fields depend on vibrations and oscillations. Einstein also maintained that everything *is* vibration, and yet, disturbed vibrations can be detrimental to our health.

It is an eye-opener to read in this fascinating book how many influences can cause us to lose sleep – how disturbed vibrations can cause disease. However, the suggestions for self-help in this book are extremely good. Both writers give advice on protecting ourselves against the detrimental influences on our energy, advice that should not be ignored. All energy, whether it be positive or negative, deserves in-depth study because I am convinced that there is so much more to learn. We should contemplate whether we use energy for our destruction or our benefit. The vital force is not *enclosed* in man, wrote Paracelsus in the sixth century, but radiates in and around him like a luminous sphere.

This energy field, or outflowing aura, reflects on all seven colours that surround us. Although we have five tangible senses, the energy fields in our life force are only used partially. If we work with energy we will see how we can develop healing within ourselves and within others where energy has been disturbed.

There are so many ways in which energy disturbances can be rectified. In kinesiology we know that muscle-testing is possible on the thymus gland. By touching the thymus gland the energy flow may be altered. Often minor manipulations can have major effects.

We must strive for balance in the five senses. There are also five types of energy necessary for happiness and these energies are all-important to a healthy life:

1. Peace of mind
2. Peace of heart
3. Peace of the body
4. Peace of the organs
5. Peace of the senses

Practice makes perfect and to achieve this we will have to practise and take exercise in the fresh air – walking, swimming and cycling. Keeping control of the muscular, the nervous and the physical systems also requires a healthy diet, supplemented by natural remedies where necessary.

NUTRITION

If we think about taste, we immediately associate this sense with food. Here I must emphasise that in order to take care of our sense of taste, we should train ourselves to be selective in what we eat and what we drink. It is said that people dig their graves with their teeth, and that man should eat to live, and not live to eat. Nutrition plays a very important role in the management of the five senses.

Many people make themselves ill by their choice of food. It is not surprising that they lose their taste when you observe them. So often I see that people do not take the time to chew their food properly and in this way the food they eat is not properly mixed with saliva, which is so necessary for a good digestion. They happily sit and force their food down without proper enjoyment, because at the same time they may be watching television or reading the newspaper.

Sometimes a short fast can be beneficial, and perhaps one day a week may be set aside for a fasting day. On such a day meals may be replaced with a glass of water, fruit or vegetable juice. In my books *How to Live a Healthy Life* and *Nature's Gift of Food* there are a number of guidelines on how to eat, how to fast, and how to improve our health by way of a good diet. We must not forget that our bodies are under severe and constant attack nowadays, not only because of some of our working practices, for example working with computers and word processors, but also, for example, by spending many hours watching television. It has been reported that Americans supposedly spend between twenty-five and forty-five hours per week watching television. This pastime not only exerts a major influence on the endocrine system, and undisputedly lowers the effectiveness of the immune system, but it most certainly affects our five senses. We must learn how best to protect ourselves and follow a more natural lifestyle. Resolve to take some exercise in the fresh air in preference to sitting motionless gazing at a television screen. It does not do to neglect our health and in order to provide for better health we must learn to relax, ensure we have sufficient sleep and combine out-of-door exercise with deep breathing exercises.

Dr Allan never tired of pointing out that congestion is the number one enemy to our health. Where congestion is present brief fasts are invaluable when combined with herbal treatment and a wholesome and healthy diet. Man lives by three forms of energy: the food we eat, the water we drink and the air we breathe. Our fluid intake is, of course, important when we consider that 65 per cent of our body is made up of fluid, while our planet consists of 75 per cent of water. In my book *Water – Healer or Poison?* I emphasise the importance of the purity of the water we drink. It may sound too simple to be true, but the quality and purity of the water we drink may indeed influence our health. There is a wide variety of spring waters available nowadays, but one of my favourites is Dee-side Springwater, which comes from Pannanich Wells in Ballater. This water contains a wealth of minerals and, in addition, has a unique substance in its biological activity which not only promotes healing but prevents illness. Professor Vincent states that water should be clean, full of oxygen, low in minerals, slightly acid and low in electrons. In Nature it is increasingly rare for all of these factors to exist at the same time in one source. Dee-side

Springwater contains all these characteristics and therefore it is considered a helpful ingredient in a healthy regime.

Another problem which influences taste is *Candida albicans*, a twentieth-century epidemic. This yeast-like fungus that is naturally present in our bodies, can become very active. Not only will it influence the brain, the nervous system, the lymphatic system, the hormones, internal organs, the muscles and joints, it will make us depressed and encourage irritable bowel syndrome (IBS), and the candida overgrowth which is often seen on the tongue will take away our sense of taste. *Candida*, as explained in my book *Viruses, Allergies and the Immune System*, is becoming more and more prevalent. Here again, one must be careful to avoid certain foods, especially yeast, wine, sugar, chocolate, mushrooms and cheese, and to help control this condition there are some very effective natural remedies available. With dietary measures and some natural remedies it is possible to bring this condition under control.

During a recent lecture I met a very gifted man, Dr Ian MacDonald, who practises in Brighton. Although we had only a little time to talk I was impressed to hear his thoughts. He observed that in a changing world, with old structures breaking down and being replaced by more holistic and humane views, while the old world crumbles, we should be prepared to shoulder our responsibilities and consider the statement of the World Health Organisation: 'Health is more than the mere absence of disease'. We must be positive about life and do whatever we can to improve our own health.

DENTAL AMALGAM – THE DANGERS

This automatically leads me to a major problem, as a result of which I have seen people's sense of taste severely affected: amalgam silver mercury fillings in our teeth. Not only has this substance robbed people of their taste sensation, it has often been detrimental to their general health and is thought, in some cases, to have led to the development of degenerative diseases. I was very happy when the other day I received news from Canada that over there pregnant mothers and kidney patients are now advised against amalgam fillings. Though suspicions have been voiced on this subject for many years, we still come across disbelief on this issue. In my own country, the Netherlands, amalgam is rarely used nowadays, and has been widely replaced by composite or other fillings that have a less dramatic effect on our health. Once again, we must all realise that we are responsible for our own health.

The other day I was heartened to see a patient whose health had greatly improved since her amalgam fillings had been replaced, and I determined to use the opportunity to mention again the potential harm to our health that can result from their use. A friendly dentist who works with me in my London clinic gave me some of his notes on this subject. He maintains that there are risks of allergies that can lead to multiple sclerosis, Parkinson's disease and kidney disease, Alzheimer's and motor neurone disease, high blood pressure, arterial insufficiency, infertility, diabetes and neuro-psychological disturbances. Please note that I am not saying that every person will have an allergic or toxic reaction to amalgam, but the evidence is growing that the symptoms of toxicity can appear within days or even thirty years later.

Amalgam consists of 53 per cent inorganic mercury, and if we consider that dental fillings are with us whether awake or asleep, and every time we use them we receive a little homoeopathic treatment, then we must recognise the amount of toxicity we are allowing to enter our bloodstream. It is important to know how we are affected by mercury intake. When we do a tongue test we see a higher rate of toxicity if the patient has a number of dental amalgam fillings. It is also interesting to see that with amalgam elimination therapies much can be done to reduce that level of toxicity.

I have studied some anamneses during consecutive visits of patients while they were gradually having their amalgam fillings replaced by fillings of a less controversial substance, and saw for myself how the toxicity levels reduced. Although it is possible for the mercury level to increase temporarily during the removal process, in the long run it is judged advisable to follow this path. In some instances, however, I occasionally advise postponing such measures until the patient has regained a better level of health. A detoxification protocol should be followed, and if you have a sympathetic dentist who is concerned about what is now considered a major health risk, he or she will advise you.

In recent years a group of dentists and scientists from Europe, Scandinavia and North America have been involved in developing a special detoxification protocol, which has proved helpful in a surprisingly large number of cases. One must not forget that mercury is a toxic substance and that it crosses all membranes, among them the blood-brain barrier; it is maintained that it even passes from the mother's fillings into the developing body of her unborn baby.

In my book *Multiple Sclerosis* I have written about this problem in considerable detail and mentioned how a great friend of mine, Dr Victor Penzer, has studied the effects of mercury for some years. When he came to Oxford University, some ten years ago, he did not receive a very friendly reception. Today, many scientists have fortunately changed their attitude to mercury and the dangers of amalgam are much more widely recognised. These dangers are that toxic and allergic reactions to amalgam or mercury can place a heavy burden on the immune system. It is believed that amalgam kills the friendly bacteria and causes varying degrees of damage throughout the entire system.

If toxicity occurs as the result of mercury, the symptoms will undoubtedly influence the immune system and reduce its effectiveness. It is impossible to consider dental amalgam as an innocuous substance. The brain is another target for mercury, one that is easily as susceptible as the immune system. I was happy to learn that the International Academy of Oral Medicine and Toxicology in Europe has advised that no one should have new amalgam fillings, and those people with amalgam fillings should follow the occasional detoxification programme. Furthermore, when existing amalgam fillings are to be replaced, a safer substance should be used.

CASE HISTORIES

Taste is as important as smell and everything possible should be done to keep our senses of smell and taste. If we are in danger of losing them, we should not leave a stone unturned to try and regain these senses. A very religious man came to see me some time ago, who told me about a biblical quotation he had often used but never understood. I had to admit that I was also familiar with the quotation: 'Oh, taste and see that the Lord is good' (Psalm 34:8). My patient explained that only now that he had regained his sense of taste did he appreciate its value. As I had deduced, he had been carrying much toxic waste material in his lymph glands and I had prescribed several potent remedies: Anthocyanidin from Nature's Best (one capsule, twice a day); CPS from Enzymatic Therapy; from Bioforce a herbal mouthwash called Dentaforce (three times daily) and garlic capsules at night. Slowly, he regained his sense of taste and that was when he explained that not until he had refound his taste had he fully understood the reference to taste in this biblical quotation. Every time he prays he now thanks the Lord for the remedies derived from Nature that restored his taste and smell. I asked him why, if he really was so grateful to God, had he not stopped smoking, because God had not created him with a chimney on his head, and I pointed out to him that smoking was a detrimental influence on his senses.

The next case history I am going to tell you is rather unusual. This concerns a 53-year-old female. This lady came to me with a hearing problem – a hissing noise and a dull ache in her head. She also told me about her total loss of taste only on the right side of her mouth. I decided to give her acupuncture and laser treatment. The following week I prescribed *Gingko biloba* (15 drops, three times daily), Emergency Essence (15 drops, twice a day), and Nicotinic Acid from Nature's Best. The latter remedy I prescribed because another name for vitamin B3 is niacin. One of the forms includes Nicotinic Acid which is closely related to nicotinamide. They all have vitamin B3 activity, but it is the 'free acid' in Nicotinic Acid that has specific effects that are associated with maintaining normal cholesterol levels in conjunction with a low-fat diet.

Nicotinic Acid functions in over fifty metabolic reactions. It plays a key role in glycolysis, reactions of the Krebs Cycle and the Hexose Monophosphate Shunt, all of which are important in the release of energy from carbohydrates. It is also needed in the deamination of amino acids, fatty acid synthesis and beta-oxydation of fatty acids.

By playing a role in the formation of red blood cells and steroids, nicotinic acid helps to maintain the general health of the body and the endocrine system. Nicotinic Acid may be chosen by people who have a moderate-to-large intake of alcohol and those with a poor protein intake. Recommended use is one capsule daily with a main meal, and it should be taken in the ratio of one part vitamin B3 as nicotinic acid and three parts of Inositol.

These three remedies helped her greatly and, when combined with acupuncture treatment, we noticed a reduction in the hissing noises, and then slowly she began to regain her sense of taste, although altogether it took several months for a marked improvement to become evident. Her story was somewhat confusing because she told me that during dental surgery some of her nerves had been cut, and I suspected that if this indeed was true, I was set an impossible task. But, fortunately, the improvement was remarkable. I still see her occasionally and she is a very much happier person.

Another case concerned a 70-year-old female patient who complained of a bad taste in her mouth. On examination of her tongue I realised that this was caused by a liver complaint. I decided to prescribe her Milk Thistle capsules, and the most potent supplement I could find was Simply Milk Thistle from Enzymatic Therapy. This is a milk thistle product standardised to contain 70 per cent of its most important natural constituents. Recommended dosage is one or two capsules three times daily as an addition to the everyday diet, or as advised by the practitioner. I also advised her to take Boldocynara from Bioforce (twice a day, ten drops after meals), as well as three garlic capsules before retiring. She too improved greatly and whenever I see her, she reassures me that her sense of taste has completely returned.

Yet another patient was a male, a dentist by profession. His case was unusual in that he had started to hyperventilate during his work. He complained that he also had lost both his senses of smell and taste, and it took me some time before I discovered that his ninth dorsal vertebra had to be corrected. This immediately relieved the hyperventilation. I also noticed that his palate was very inflamed and he told me that often the chewing of food was accompanied by soreness. It was strange that even though he faithfully followed my advice, there was little or no change in his condition. However, as well as recommending some natural remedies, I suggested some breathing exercises, and this seemed to be beneficial. The remedies I recommended were Dr Vogel's Echinaforce (20 drops, three times daily before meals), Concentration Essence from the Flower Essences, and finally a remedy called Oral Basics Supplement from Enzymatic Therapy, which provides a combination of nutrients and herbs to support healthy gum tissue. The anti-oxidant activity of vitamins A, C and E help to neutralise damaging free radicles that may affect gum tissue. Calcium and boron are required for healthy teeth and bones. Glucosamine sulphate, the most absorbable form of glucosamine, plays a key role in connective tissue function. Extracts of hawthorn berry and bilberry are rich in flavonoids, which are important for strong collagen structure. The recommended dosage for Oral Basics Supplement is as before, one or two tablets taken three times daily, as an addition to the everyday diet, or as advised by the practitioner.

A girl in her early twenties explained that she would lose her sense of taste for an entire day, yet be aware of a very unpleasant taste in her mouth. During the examination I asked her if it were at all possible that she was pregnant, which she denied. I suggested that she went to see her general practitioner who, after the appropriate tests, confirmed that she was indeed pregnant. However, her problem still persisted. Although she was quite happy about the news of her pregnancy, she still wanted to get rid of the unpleasant taste in her mouth. This we managed to overcome with the help of Enzymatic Therapy's Gingerall, an encapsulated remedy, standardised to contain an unprecedented 20 per cent total pungent compounds, calculated as 6-ginerol and 6-shogaol. Research shows this percentage makes Gingerall the most potent standardised ginger extract available. The ginger oil in Gingerall has also been shown to be of great value in the treatment of hay fever and other allergic complaints.

4

Hearing

Sometimes I have listened with interest to people voicing their personal opinions about whether it would be worse to be blind or to be deaf. Invariably their opinion would be formed by their own situation, or by situations of which they had inside knowledge. I can only assume that either condition is very difficult to cope with and I am grateful that I will never be put in the position of having to make such a choice. If we think about it, it does not take long to realise how dependent a deaf person is on his or her senses in order to understand what is going on by studying people's facial expressions, their eyes, their mouth, or their gestures. It cannot be easy, but it is encouraging to see how, by experience, a deaf or partially deaf person usually manages to cope quite well. The fact, however, that they may have learned to live with their disability does not alter the fact that, given a choice, they would always admit that their dearest wish would be to regain their hearing. In this context it should be remembered that it is not always a hopeless situation because, depending on the cause of their disability, it may be possible to reverse the process.

When a person becomes aware that his or her ability to hear is gradually diminishing, it should never be left to chance. I am a great believer in trying everything possible and leaving no stone unturned in trying to overcome whatever the condition may be.

The ear has two functions: to hear and to provide balance. Both functions are very precious and highly sensitive. Unfortunately, both functions are also easily disturbed, and when I hear people remark that they sometimes clean out their ears with a hairpin, or with other hard or sharp objects, I cringe with apprehension and immediately warn them against the dangers of poking in the ear with such objects. The ear is not only a wonderfully developed organ, but also extremely sensitive to interference. Vibrations can easily upset the sense of hearing, as will be confirmed by many people who travel regularly by air. Only too often they require medical help in order to restore their diminished hearing ability.

In order for us to be able to hear, the delicate nerve endings in the cochlea must be stimulated. The brain performs a major role in supporting our capacity to hear, sending the messages we receive as speech, noise, music and sounds of all kinds. Of the passages that originate in the middle ear, one is destined for the mastoid process, while the other leads to the Eustachian tube, ending in the nose. We often find that a blockage of the Eustachian tubes results in discomfort, and the change in pressure experienced while flying is more than capable of releasing pulp that can settle on a semi-permanent basis in these tubes. A catarrhal or fungal condition can also be the cause of such a blockage.

The inner ear, which contains all the nerve endings, is responsible for detecting fluid, while the semi-circular canals are the organs of balance. If we keep moving the fluid against the nerve endings it will stimulate messages to the brain. All kinds of problems can happen to the ear in this very delicate process. I have been in practice for more than thirty-five years and at times I have been utterly shocked by some of the conditions I have been asked to treat. When the cause of the condition is beyond the individual's control I fully sympathise, but I find it harder to accept some of the dire effects which can be ascribed to negligence.

One of the first senses is touch, and this is often also explained as balance. Many people experience balancing problems because something in the ear is not as it should be. I have found that general balance problems may be overcome with the aid of *Gingko biloba* (fifteen drops, taken three times daily).

Figure 12: Cross-section of the ear

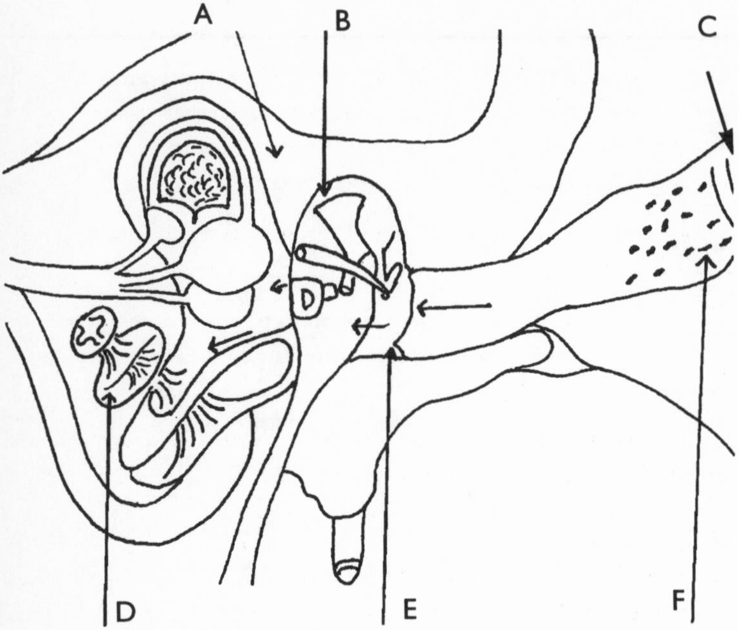

A – Additional sound path
If the eardrum or the middle ear have been injured, they can be bypassed by sending sound vibration to the inner ear through the bones of the skull.

B – Middle Ear
Sends sound waves to inner ear over chain of three bones: the hammer, anvil, and stirrup. They magnify sound; are the smallest bones in the body.

C – Outer Ear
Catches sound waves and directs them into the ear canal. Ridges of

outer ear help keep water and perspiration from going into interior of the ear.

D – Inner Ear
Contains the cochlea, a snail-shaped bone. Tiny nerve cells in the cochlea send vibrations over the auditory nerve to the brain. Hearing then results.

E – Eardrum
Acts as drumhead to pick up sound vibrations and send them to middle ear. No larger than the pupil of your eye, it is thinner than tissue paper.

F – Ear Canal
Leads to inside of the ear. It is about a quarter-inch long and the size of a lead pencil. Arrows indicate path which sound waves follow in the ear.

We cannot fail to wonder why hearing problems have become so much more common nowadays. Could it indeed be, as the World Health Organisation (WHO) maintains, that noise has such a detrimental influence? WHO claims that noise is a significant cause of fatigue. Acoustic engineers working for WHO have identified the key frequency ranges to which the human body is most sensitive and have developed over fifteen noise barriers to insulate these. This clearly indicates that noise is recognised as a major health hazard.

With this in mind we have an obligation to protect ourselves and avoid the possibility of causing permanent damage to our hearing. Manufacturers of motorised and electrical equipment are increasingly aware of these dangers and concentrate on reducing the noise levels in their designs. Today's noise-reducing factors have become sales features in marketing campaigns for motor cars, washing machines and sound equipment, to name but a few products.

It is also important to bear in mind that allergies, viruses, parasites and bacterial influences must be treated at an early stage. For example, streptococcus bacteria can result not only in tonsillitis, but this same bacteria can also affect the hearing. Allergic reactions can also result in a hearing deficiency.

Tension is often the cause of vibrational disturbances in hearing. We often find when treating a patient with cranial osteopathy that tension can be relieved by working on the endocrine zones and at the same time the patient's hearing is likely to improve. This was clearly demonstrated during a recent treatment session, when my patient suddenly looked up and with an expression of pleasant surprise, mixed with delight, remarked that he felt he could hear better. This frequently occurs during osteopathic treatment, because the skull and the facial bones may have moved out of position and if the treatment is designed to move these back into place – in other words to restore the balance – a speedy improvement in the hearing may be brought about.

The bones of the skull may have moved out of position for many reasons. First consider the jawbone: if the left side of the skull is low, the right side is forced to rise out of position. This causes the teeth on the left side of the mouth to close much more firmly than on the right side, and then we are inclined to chew our food on the left side of our mouth. By doing this we take the pressure off the teeth on the right side, which will restrict the nerve action and the circulation of the blood to both the upper and lower teeth on that side of the face. In many cases this is the cause of ulcers of the gums, toothache or pyorrhoea. If the lower jawbone is low, then the cheekbone will also be lower. This causes the sinus and facial bone to twist out of position. By standing before a mirror and placing one finger of the right hand under the right cheekbone and one finger of the left hand under the left cheekbone, we can tell just how much the facial bones have moved out of position. Now this unnatural pressure of the facial bones will cause trouble in the antrums and the adenoids, and will cause a blockage in the sinuses.

In a close examination of the bones of your face, one eye will often appear to be lower than the other. This is the case when the facial bones are out of position. Then the frontal or forehead bone will show the same indication; thus moving the bone of the forehead down on the left side causes the left eye to be lower. As the left side of the frontal part of the skull moves downward, it naturally causes the back of the skull on the same side to move upward. This will interfere with the position of your mastoid gland, exerting an unnatural pressure on the medulla and interfering with your sight and hearing, as it causes the mastoid bone to rise, corresponding with the back of the skull. This movement will prevent the head from being in a straight position upon the atlas (the top bone of the spine), impinging upon the nerves of the spine and causing a lack of energy in the brain, eyes, ears, nose and throat. Thus, to a certain extent, the circulation is cut off to the different parts of the head and face.

In many cases people who are unsteady on their feet will occasionally misstep and fall or turn their ankle, this being caused by pressure on the brain. Again, there are people who at times stagger, or are afraid to climb a ladder to unreasonable heights, or to look down from the top of high buildings, because they feel dizzy. The cause of all this interference is located in the brain directly under the temporal bone, which is just above the ear. The left side of the forehead being low results in pressure on this bone, crowding it in, in turn bringing pressure to bear on the brain. This same bone on the opposite side of the head will protrude, causing a fullness on the right side of the head, all this in turn executing pressure on the centre of balance in the brain. This pressure not only causes the above troubles, but it also unbalances the entire system of thinking, will and the action of the entire body.

If the skull is higher on one side than the other, it will cause a pressure on the brain, stopping the function of this portion of the brain and the nervous system that connects with some of the vital parts of our body. In many cases the skull moving out of position is responsible for the appearance of lymphatic tumours in the scalp.

If the forehead is out of alignment, one side higher than the other, you will readily notice it in the bony structure above the eyes. If there is a depression in the skull, just behind the forehead, it will cause the neck to become stiff, the shoulders to move out of alignment, and trouble will arise in the hands and wrists.

On each side of the top centre of the skull, there is a direct connection between the underlying portion of the brain and the feet, especially the toes and metatarsal arches.

If a defect appears in the back of the skull, we may have trouble with both eyes and ears. These misplaced bones of the skull exert pressure on the brain or the cells of the brain connected with different parts of our body.

Consider the misplaced sections of the skull and the great influence and pressure that they will cause on the nerves and circulation of the head and face, and the pressure that is brought to bear on different sections of the brain. It may take a number of treatments to restore the skull to a perfect condition and relieve the nerves and the circulation of the red blood.

The mastoid bones, or process, are located just behind the ears and continue back along the base of the skull. They lie between the temporal and occipital bones. As with the other divisions of the skull, they sometimes move out of position and cause considerable hearing problems. If the left side of the skull moves forward, it will interfere with the hearing of the left ear, causing considerable trouble with dry wax. We may find the same disturbance on the right side of the skull and ear.

Ordinarily, we do not pay much attention to the mastoid bones, but we should not underestimate their importance, as inside them we find air chambers similar to the sinuses in the frontal part of the head. The interior of the lower part of the mastoid bones consists of small cells resembling those of a honeycomb. These cells contain marrow and hormones of different kinds which provide lubrication for the ear. Later it becomes a waxy substance. In cases where the red blood is interfered with, or there is a lack of circulation, the heat ratio in the mastoids and ears will decrease. The shell, or the outside of the mastoid bones, will become almost as hard as ivory.

The mastoids play an important role in our hearing. The two mastoid bones are connected by tissue. This tissue extends forward making a connection with the inner eardrum. The outer eardrums, right and left, connect with the mastoid glands, which are directly behind them. These glands are not as noticeable in children as they are in older people. If there is an interference in the ears caused by the mastoid glands, our senses of sight, taste and smell will be affected. In cases where the skull is deformed or out of order, it will bring pressure to bear on the mastoid glands, interfering with the medulla, and also affecting the senses of taste and smell. The seat of sight is located in the back of the head near the mastoid bone. If there is unnatural pressure on this bone, it will diminish our ability to see.

In many cases of inflammation in the mastoid bone, a fever may develop. This causes a soreness of the bone behind the ear causing an enlargement of the mastoid glands and interfering with the tongue and throat. One gland from each mastoid extends down the throat and attaches to the collarbone. A feverish condition of the mastoid may result in many disorders and throat trouble, causing large deposits of phlegm or mucus in the throat. You may recognise these conditions by a very bad odour in the nostrils. There is another connection with the mastoid – a small acute gland travelling upwards close behind the ear. This has been referred to as an inferior duct and in many cases has been surgically removed. However, the removal of this little gland or duct may cause serious trouble in the brain, as blood poisoning sometimes develops in the mastoid. The position of the back of the skull has a strong influence over the mastoid and glands.

Every organ of the body will indicate its condition by a symptom. When there is trouble in the eyes, ears, throat, etc., you will find cold spots on the head, the back of the neck, the shoulders and arms, and superficially above the location area of each organ of the body. For each organ of the body perspires as does the forehead, and if for any reason the perspiration is checked, a cold spot develops. If the liver is not working properly, there will be a cold spot over the liver as the action of the sweat glands will have ceased. As the perspiration leaves the body in other areas, you will notice a peculiar odour that signifies the retarded action of the liver. At other times, the odour of the body may be like that of the stomach or bowels, or like that of the kidneys after an action.

You can locate for yourself the cause of the trouble by passing the palms of the hands over the skin. When you come to a cold spot, you will know that the organ beneath needs attention. If the gall-bladder is impaired, or the gall-duct, you will find the cold spot located on the right side of your body just at the bottom of the diaphragm near the bottom of the ribs. Your spleen is also of importance. You will find the cold spot for the pancreas and the spleen on the opposite side of the body – on the left side – just at the bottom of the ribs.

If the cause of your distress is in breathing or in the respiratory system, then right at the end of the breast bone you will find the solar plexus, which will take care of your breathing for you in a very short time. You must understand that this greatest nerve centre of the body, called a plexus, connects groups of nerves extending to all organs of the body, and when you treat this centre, you will immediately feel the warmth of the minerals passing through your body, into each and every organ.

Our thinking faculties are divided into three separate parts: objective, subjective and subconscious. Our thinking is transferred from the universal mind to the three divisions of our brain. Our thought, action and deeds depend greatly upon the action of our conscious system, and upon our brain. If the organism of our body is not functioning properly, it interferes with the communications from the conscious system in our brains, causing heavy, sluggish thinking. A torpid liver, gall-bladder trouble, constipation and many other ailments interfere with the consciousness and detract from the action of the brain. In this study of brain, mind and thought, we will see many different bodily influences that can and will interfere with our thinking.

Various parts of our body have a direct connection with the brain. Thus, a disarranged skull may interfere with any natural talent that humanity is entitled to exercise. If the temple division of the skull is out of position, it is easily detected by moving your hands slowly over the skull and you will discover a groove or uneven surface of the skull. If the parietal bones bulge on either side, this will cause pressure on the nervous system of the entire body, causing the individual to worry or experience fear. If the frontal bones have moved far enough out of position to cause pressure on the frontal part of the brain, this will interfere with the intelligence. If the lower division of the skull in the back of the head (occipital) moves downward the slightest bit, it will exert pressure on the mastoid gland and this will interfere with the hearing. This same condition may cause serious eye strain. Now, if these pressures are brought to bear on the different parts of the brain, it causes interference with our thinking.

In order to have clear action, we must have a clear brain. In order to have a clear brain, we must have a body that is functioning properly, free from aches and pains, free from constipation and indigestion. Our lymphatic system must work efficiently. The flesh and skin must carry out their duties without interference. Our conscious system must be free from depression, and our liver, gall-bladder, pancreas and spleen must function properly. We must have unity between our body, our soul and our spirit. Then we can think correctly, both physically and spiritually. We should be very careful when we are translating the mind into thought and action.

ACUPUNCTURE

Many experiments have been done in relation to acupuncture of the ear, particularly with the aim of establishing precise points of location for treatments.

The Russians reported some clinical experiments made in 1959–61 elaborating on methods and research done in 1900–50. Doctor Nogier of France claimed to have discovered an analogy between the ear zones and other parts of the body – their hypersensibility being via the trigeminal nerve to the ear, the neck and the spinal nerves all having communication to and with the vago-sympathetic.

Painful points are searched for in the ear by means of the special probe. Having determined the painful point or points, these are marked and then cleansed with some spirit, then the instrument is used or applied with slight pressure on these painful areas.

The external ear contains all the visceral reflexes which are significant for the glands, including the endocrine glands. Care and gentleness is therefore required in locating the points because they are so minute.

This can be likened to small projections of the spinal column as in reflex therapy. The lobe of the ear corresponds to the eyes. Hence it is not merely a superstition when gypsies pierce their lobes, claiming benefit to their eyes.

A Dr Nada of Parma once reported a man being stung in the ear by a bee or wasp. He reacted by trembling in the lower leg and sole of the foot, resulting in him being temporarily unable to walk. The cause of this reaction was that the fibre of the acoustic vagus nerve also passes via the intercostal vagus to the sciatic nerve.

If you study the external ear as depicted in *Gray's Anatomy* you will see the resemblance of the human ear to the embryo (foetus) on its head and representing the whole body. If you turn the diagram upside down the resemblance will be even more apparent.

In certain sections these points of correspondence are arranged in an anatomical, harmonious and logical manner. In other sections can be found the function of the glands and in the centre is the association with connective tissue. The head of the embryo or foetus is indicated by the anti-(outer) helix.

If one follows the anti-helix upward one finds the spinal equivalent. The coccyx is found at the junction of the anti-helix under the rim of the ear. The anti-helix embodies the spine, dividing the auricle into two different parts. The hollow shell is surrounded, into which the horizontal helix root fixes itself.

The shell contains points for all the internal organs. At the root is the diaphragm of the foetus and in the upper part the abdominal organs. In the lower part are the thoracic organs as well as the regions for the endocrine glands. In this lower part is the external meatus, which is covered by the tragus. Between the tragus and anti-tragus is a zone which contains a larger number of points acting on the endocrine glands.

There is a longitudinal groove between the helix and anti-helix which would expand to the upper rim of the ear. In this part are arranged the shoulder, the arm and the wrist joint further upward.

The proximity of the ovaries and the forehead points explains the occurrence of migraines and nervous disturbances during the menstrual periods. The point acting on the heart lies close to the thyroid gland.

The whole of the organism can be influenced by gentle massage with the probe. This should be carried out for not more than two minutes in each ear. According to the pressure used, harmony can be achieved.

In certain cases, where the energy and its circulation are too strong, sedating the points as indicated could be carried out by placing the point of the probe on the tender point and applying gentle pressure.

Dr Gardes examined the whole auricle in an asthma patient and in the lower segment he found a tender spot. The pituitary gland point was also found to be tender. The probe was placed on these points in each ear and within a few minutes the patient felt better and the spasm subsided.

The reflex points in the ear have proved very useful for both mental and congenital disorders. Even cases of rheumatism that developed after childbirth, when treated, showed great improvement.

Many people have a built-in phobia about the use of needles – sometimes with adverse effects. Recent research has proved that the treatment is just as effective with the use of the special probe.

MAGNETIC THERAPIES

Instead of using acupuncture I have also obtained good results, especially when treating younger people, by using copper and zinc magnets. The ability to treat with magnets is not a new concept. The Greek physician Galen researched magnetism as far back as 200 BC and through the ages dedicated seekers of perfection in healing have contributed their findings on the healing power of the magnet. Scientists have proved that the human body is a source of energy, and measurement of the ion currents of the heart and brain have been carried out by magneto-cardiogram and magneto-encephalogram.

Much has been written elsewhere about magnets and energy fields and I do not propose to give a dissertation on the science of magnetism but simply to highlight those facts which are most relevant to healing.

Magnetism governs the universe: all planets transmit magnetic emanations and the earth is surrounded by its own magnetic fields which project magnetic energy to all living organisms. The human body itself is a magnet and is a receiver for incoming electromagnetic energies. We are all aware that the moon affects the tides, as does the sun. When the energies of the moon and sun are aligned, their combined pull upon the earth results in abnormally high tides. Man is also affected by these gravitational forces, which can cause changes in the physical, mental and biochemical functions of the body.

Magnetism affects every cell in the body and a magnetic field can exert a direct influence upon the thalamencephalon which controls the endocrine system. It can be demonstrated that the endocrine system acts upon the muscular system which, in turn, exerts a controlling influence upon the skeletal system. The skeletal system, especially the spine, controls and provides protection to the central nervous system and so we see the pattern emerging.

Taking the whole of the human electrical biomagnetic system into consideration, the brain must be looked upon as a computer which conveys sensations along the nerve fibres stimulating electrical impulses which send instructions to the other parts of the body.

Blood plays an important part in the human body and magnetic force affects the body through the circulatory system. A magnet applied to the body sends a weak current through the blood and the quantity of ions is increased, thus benefiting the circulation. Experiments have been carried out where the fluids and plasma are separated from the red blood cells. When the red blood cells are placed on a slide under a microscope, and a magnet is held under the slide, these red blood cells will spin round to point in one direction. This represents the alignment of iron and ions. When any form of energy is aligned, the result is a harnessing of a high level of energy.

Various other experiments have established that the South Pole of the magnet is positive and the North Pole is negative. North Pole energy reduces and dissolves, whereas South Pole energy increases and expands.

I repeat that magnetic therapy is not new. Homoeopaths are aware of the healing properties of magnets and the well-known homoeopathic author Dr Allan extensively covered three remedies prepared from the magnet: *Magnetis Polus Ambo, Magnetis Polus Acticus* and *Magnetis Polis Australis.*

During the last two decades magnetic therapies have gained wider recognition and the practice of this therapy is increasing worldwide. The type of magnetic therapy most commonly used involves placing magnets on the most painful areas of the body, and in cases where there is no local pain, magnets are applied to the extremities.

The British Biomagnetic Association has been formed to introduce a technique which combines the philosophy of acupuncture with some of the principles of magnetic energy. Consider for a moment the theory of ionisation. Scientists interested in genetic mechanics and chemistry discovered that every cell in the body had, as it were, two small factories – one working to produce acid and the other alkaline. Providing the production of acid and alkaline was balanced in a four-hour period, they neutralised each other and in so doing released energy. All naturopaths know that bacteria, viruses and every minute organism which affects the human organism is either acid- or alkaline-based, and the scientists who discovered genetic ionisation realised that if a disease affecting a particular organ or set of cells was acid-based, the bacteria would die naturally if the cells could be given an alkaline wash. Unfortunately, it is not possible to do this with modern chemistry. It is possible, however, to achieve this by using acupuncture and magnets: substitute yang for acid and yin for alkaline and you have the theory of ionisation, discovered by the Chinese some 5,000 years ago.

There are a number of methods by which the optimum pH value or balancing of ions can be achieved, needles and moxibustion being the most frequently used. If, however, the swing of the pH has settled predominantly in one field, i.e. in diseases such as rheumatoid arthritis, rheumaticus deformens, polyarthritis, cancer or diabetes, where the balance is predominantly alkaline, there will be too much disturbance for either needles or moxibustion to correct the imbalance and it is here that the application of biomagnetic therapy can be of value through exerting a greater gravitational force.

This is by no means the only application for biomagnetic therapy and to illustrate this I include two diverse examples below.

151

A young woman was involved in a motor-cycle accident. The humerus was completely smashed; bone surgery and bone grafts had left the elbow completely bent and a spur had grown causing extreme pain. The spur was reduced surgically but her pain increased. As a last resort the surgeon prescribed morphia-based tablets which resulted in a weight loss of three stones and inability to sleep due to pain. The concentration she required for her studies was totally lacking and the young woman became suicidal. Eventually she decided to seek help from an alternative practitioner. Magnets were placed along the scar and on selected acupoints. Her treatment lasted approximately thirty minutes. Within six hours she telephoned to say that the pain had reduced dramatically and the following morning she reported complete freedom from pain. That was six months ago and there has been no recurrence of her pain.

A boy aged 13 was a chronic asthmatic and a very severe case. He was on steroids which were causing him to swell and retain fluid and a diuretic was prescribed to reduce the amount of fluid. Those in the field will appreciate that it is not possible to use acupuncture to treat a patient who is on steroids. The boy was gradually taken off steroids and given the first treatment; again magnets were applied to specific acupoints, the treatment lasting from twenty-five to thirty minutes. On the day of his next appointment his mother telephoned to say that because of transport difficulties she was unable to bring him for his second treatment but that he was so much better that it was unbelievable. For a variety of reasons we did not see the boy for a further six weeks, but I did hear of him.

Once a year in this lad's part of the world there is a 26-mile marathon and, incredible as it may seem, this boy entered. He ran the whole course, coming in last but one! His mother tells me that he has not had an asthmatic attack since.

Of course, not all cases are as remarkable as these two, but the percentage of complete and speedy recovery is very high. In many instances strategically placed magnets obviate the necessity for skeletal manipulation, needles and homoeopathy. Biomagnetic therapy is gaining in popularity and is usually regarded as all-embracing and almost totally holistic.

The basic concept of biomagnetic therapy incorporates the application of specially designed magnets, made of rare earth metal with a gold and aluminium insert, to specific key points on the eight extraordinary meridians. These meridians have a common meeting place in the thalamus which, as mentioned earlier, controls the sympathetic and parasympathetic nervous system, endocrine system, muscular system, skeletal and central nervous systems.

Every day of our lives we are subjected to the effects of magnetic energy. Magnetic energy is in fact a force field that results when an electron moves, rather than energy. Even as you read this, you are creating magnetic fields and, likewise, are subject to their effects. This flow of electrons is considered to exist from the North Pole to the South Pole and vice versa. In the three-dimensional context there exists another pole: the neutral pole. This neutral pole is not unlike the equator that exists between the North and South Poles of the earth. At this pole there is no magnetic force, but a neutral state.

Many phenomena in this world exist because of the force field surrounding moving particles. Studies have shown that the association of a natural magnetic phenomenon gives rise to inferior or superior health, depending upon the force field. The art of 'witching' for water, likewise, involves magnetic energy flows.

Horticulturists were among the first to investigate the properties of magnetism. Early in the 1940s, work with time-lapse photography showed that certain plants, in order to bloom, required well-defined periods of light and darkness. The light that we experience is the result of movement of electrons and other particles. Hence, visible light is an electromagnetic spectrum. Plants have been made to grow faster and stronger with the aid of standard bar magnets. The use of magnetic fields will reduce the time period from planting to marketing for flowering plants, especially indoor varieties.

EAR INFECTIONS
Chronic ear infections affect 20–40 per cent of children under the age of six and account for more than half of all visits to

paediatricians. This has been conservatively estimated. The standard medical approach to ear infections in children is to prescribe antibiotics and/or antihistamines. If the ear infection is of a long-standing duration, and does not respond to drugs, surgery is often involved. It is sad when surgery takes place, and although this only requires a tiny plastic tube into the eardrum that helps drain fluid into the throat via the Eustachian tube, it still is a major intervention for small children. The procedure is known as myringotomy. It is not a curative procedure, but it does sometimes prevent further ear infections. Recurrent ear infection is sometimes associated with bottle-feeding. It appears that in children who were breast-fed this is a less common complaint. Cow's milk contains nine times more protein than mother's milk, and this is thought to be an influence. Moreover, it is widely accepted that breast-feeding is likely to prevent food allergies, particularly if the mother avoids sensitising foods during pregnancy.

Since a child's digestive tract is quite permeable to food antigens, especially during the first three months, careful control of eating patterns is necessary. It has been established that allergies are a major cause of chronic ear infections. Studies reported in the *American Journal of Natural Medicine* show that 85–90 per cent of children with ear infections have allergies: 16 per cent to inhalants, 40 per cent to certain foods and 70 per cent to both. Other studies have shown that allergic reactions can easily result in a recurring otitis media, which is a middle ear infection. Most allergies were to cow's milk, with wheat taking second place, as well as varying degrees of allergic reactions to cheese, corn, peanuts, chicken, tomatoes and apples, to name but a few. This more or less bears out my own experience, because I have come across this in my own practice all too frequently. Acute infections can often be controlled with a high dose of Echinaforce – for young children ten drops, twice a day, and perhaps twice this dosage for adults. To this may be added one capsule of Phytobiotic for young children; again double the dosage for adults.

If children display a restless nature the homoeopathic remedy *Aconite* 30 will be helpful and in the case of pain, *Pulsatilla* 6 is recommended. Special care should be taken if children like swimming, in which case zinc or vitamin B supplement should then be considered as an extra safeguard.

Yet another problem might be the cause when a gradual hearing loss is recognised: otosclerosis, which is a common cause of deafness in adults. This can develop at a very slow and gradual pace, and is therefore often barely noticed. The remedy to use in such instances is *Gingko biloba* (fifteen drops, twice daily). Severe cases often benefit from an extra boost by adding to this one capsule of *Gingko Phytosome*, a product from Enzymatic Therapy, twice a day. It goes without saying that in the case of a gradual hearing impairment the ears should be checked for the presence of wax. Three drops of Eucalyptus oil on a piece of cotton-wool can be used to clear blocked ears. To this I want to add a word of caution with respect to the advice sometimes given by aromatherapists. In cases of chronic earache, when it may be suggested that a few drops of slightly heated almond oil be dropped in the ears, I would advise against this.

I have always found the Bioforce remedy Plantago very helpful. This is a fresh herb preparation recommended for serious coughing and congestion, as well as chronic inflammation of the mucous membranes of the lungs. Its specific properties are also beneficial for earache and toothache. I usually prescribe ten drops twice a day; at the same time I recommend placing a piece of cotton-wool sprinkled with a few drops of Plantago deep in the ear. In cases of minor deafness or earache this will be of great help, especially once the ear has become blocked. In such instances relief can also be obtained with one or two drops of St John's wort in the ear.

I remember one of the nurses in my clinic in the Netherlands who complained about painful earache which she seemed unable to overcome. I advised her to chop a fresh onion, wrap this in a piece of linen and place this on the ear as a compress. She was to cover this with a hot, damp towel and keep it in place for about half an hour. Within twenty minutes she called to tell me that a lot of foul matter had been discharged from her ear, and how much better she already felt. She could hardly believe that this was all due to such an old-fashioned remedy as a chopped onion. This remedy can also be successfully applied in the case of *Otitis externa*, together with two tablets of *Hepar sulph.* D4 daily. For middle ear infections – *Otitis media* – I would prescribe Echinaforce, an outstanding natural antibiotic, but if the ear is suppurating medical advice should be sought immediately.

In the case of an ear infection caused by staphylococcus aureus or streptococcus beta haemolyticus, *Plantago lanceolata* is very helpful. For red and swollen ears take ten drops of *Apis* D4 three times daily, while for an acute middle ear infection *Belladonna* D4 is recommended. For children, if they have an earache as the result of a cold or flu, give them ten drops of Chamomile D4 three times a day. If the Eustachian tube is infected, *Ferrum phosphoricum* D12 (one tablet every two hours) will be beneficial.

TINNITUS AND MÉNIÈRE'S DISEASE

It seems that nowadays more and more people suffer from tinnitus. Some people complain about rushing noises in the ears, while others complain about high-pitched or whistling sounds. Tinnitus is an extremely debilitating condition, which can be caused by chronic catarrh or a fungal growth, or occasionally by a musculo-skeletal problem in the neck. If the latter is the case manipulation may be helpful. There is still insufficient medical knowledge on the subject, but there is no doubt how severely this disease can affect people. It is worth remembering that tinnitus can often be helped by acupuncture, and even though I have heard a great many people claim that they are too scared to even consider trying acupuncture treatment, they should understand that if this treatment is provided by well-qualified practitioners, there is no reason to fear discomfort or pain.

Basically, acupuncture begins with a diagnosis of the individual's energy imbalance, because such an imbalance is highly likely, especially with ear problems, and this is why acupuncture is helpful. The stimulation of different areas, affecting the right acupuncture point, with a pulse associated, informs the practitioner about the energy of the organ. The practitioner will then make his or her diagnosis and decide which acupuncture points are relevant in the treatment. I can assure you that this is a most effective method for treating tinnitus. Often the fresh extract of *Gingko biloba* together with *Gingko Phytosome* will help, sometimes combined with Niacin B3, depending on the severity of the condition and the practitioner's opinion.

Ménière's disease is more difficult to treat and as well as acupuncture, manipulation may be required. Moreover, patients with this condition usually react well to the *Petasites* extract. Usually this treatment is also considered suitable for vertigo. The exact cause of Ménière's disease is still not known, but it is widely considered to be a disorder of a recurrent prostrating vertigo. Sensory hearing loss and tinnitus is usually associated with a dilation of the membranous labyrinth. The attacks of vertigo in Ménière's disease can last from a few to twenty-four hours and many people often reach the point of despair during such attacks. One of my patients, an elderly lady, admitted that she had bought herself a 'Walkman' for no other reason than to play music in order to drown out the other sounds that reverberated through her head during some of these attacks.

If you seek advice from your GP you will most likely be referred to an ear, nose and throat specialist. Not so long ago I saw a patient in my clinic with acute mastoiditis, who had not been prepared to consult a doctor, and this patient was certainly suffering greatly because of her stubbornness. Recently I also saw a lady who came to see me twenty-four hours after a dental appointment. She informed me that during an extraction at the dentist the previous day, she heard a noise in her ear. In the afternoon she returned to the dentist to speak to him about this, but unfortunately the dentist was unable to help her. Hence she arrived at my clinic to seek help and during my examination I realised that her TM joint – temporo-mandibular joint – was out of place. I could reassure her that I have seen quite a number of patients with this condition. An impairment of the TM joint can lead to considerable muscle dysfunction and over the years I have treated people for sciatica when I discovered that their jaw was out of place. To come back to the lady who had such an unfortunate experience during her visit to the dentist, I can reassure you that with manipulation I succeeded in rectifying the TM joint, with the result that the sounds in her head disappeared completely.

Very often, when the TM joint is out of place it presses on the hyoid. This may not only affect the sciatic nerve – the longest in the body – but the vagus nerve may easily be impaired as well. The vagus nerve is often described as the life nerve of the human body. It controls the force and rate of the heart. When it is stimulated, it slows the heart, strengthening its force and action, giving more time for the body to repair the body, so to speak. It overcomes sympathetic nervous tension and muscle contraction almost immediately. The vagus nerve acts as a good and reliable brake to the sympathetic nervous system. It also activates the viscera. Its para-sympathetic fibres are predominant in all glands of internal secretion. It activates the peristaltic movement of the gastro-intestinal tract, and it promotes elimination of uric acid by activating the kidneys, lungs and excretory glands.

The vagus nerve is truly the master builder. Its tools are the internal secretory glands, which is the reason for such quick and miraculous responses being obtained through its stimulation or relaxation.

ZONE THERAPY USING THE FEET

Let us return to the feet here and look in greater detail at how they can be used to treat imbalances. A zone chart of the feet would show clear marking of all the organs, as well as the zones. These have been tested from time to time. Sometimes practitioners have differed as to the exact location of the various organs, but going into detail of the zones of the body, these parts are near enough accurate. In most heart problems you will find that the solar plexus is involved and relaxing treatment of this area will give good results.

The big toe seems a very important indicator. Often a joint is displaced or a bunion present. These can ultimately cause head trouble. The big toe represents the head itself. The pituitary and pineal glands are placed in such a way that the other toes are really the faculties of the head.

Life generally consists of three principles:

1. The *Going* principle is usually associated with the hips and gluteals.
2. The shoulders are associated with the *Doing* principle.

3. The head, of course, is the *Thinking* principle.

These three principles can be applied to the zones in the body.

Besides these principles we also have the three body states: according to Indian folklore and medicine, the fluids of the body were accounted for by the emotional state, and all bones and hard tissue were held to be allied to the spiritual state.

The glands are clearly shown on the feet. There is also another very important organ called the diaphragm. This separates the lower regions of elimination from the upper regions of assimilation. Looking for calluses and corns can give us a clear picture of the state of the body – if there are any of these on the underside of the foot near the lung area, it could very well tell us the quality of life within the frame and thus point to the state of the nervous system as well.

The liver area is very important as it is the area of human action and activity. If this is congested it shows in our moods and mental state. How often have we heard it said that a person is liverish, just because he is in a mood or out of sorts?

The solar plexus, as already mentioned, is often the area to contact for heart trouble. It is known as the centre of the yoga chakras or gland area. It acts to balance the above with the below. It usually becomes tense in times of stress and in cases of frustration or emotional upsets. Always remember that stress shows in the feet as the negative and lowest point in the body. Treating the zones on the feet really treats the person and not the ailment as what is involved is in fact a reflex from the body. The body currently travels to all reflex areas.

The study of the physiology and mechanics of the feet will give you a good pointer. A person with fallen arches (longitudinal arch) will have less spring and ease in his movement, and this will point to trouble with the intestines. The metatarsal arch is usually reflected in the nervous system, and reflects the lack of life force and internal stress.

The nails can show up many defects, as these are usually a reflex to the head. Where they appear unhealthy, this indicates that there is a continual struggle going on within the body. Similarly, corns and calluses show up as stress patterns on the areas affected. These cause further pressures on the feet and, like a vicious circle, it goes from bad to worse.

The feet perspire heavily during the stage of adolescence. Bunions indicate the individual's quality of life possessed at the time. These are the little pointers that will set you thinking for yourself. As a general guide to the glands, I shall give you the locations as I have found them to affect the glandular areas:

- The pineal gland coincides with the upper medial corner of the big toenail.
- The pituitary coincides with the lower medial corner of the nail of the big toe.
- The throat or thyroid coincides with the lower part of the neck of the big toe.
- The solar plexus is situated at the lower medial edge of the ball of the foot.
- The gonads or genitals are situated where the two heel surfaces meet medially.
- The anal or coccyx is located at the bottom of the heel.
- The navel is situated at the waist level of the feet.

What really happens when you work on the areas of the feet? You are really working on the parts of the body concerned. Actually, you are helping to loosen up the molecular structure, so that the cells of the body are allowed a breathing space.

The glandular areas are all functional and represent the quality of life which flows from the head, down to the lowest or anal centre. In fact, the loosening of these glandular areas affects the upper areas with the lower areas – the positive with the negative principle. This is further enhanced with the use of the hands, which represent the neutral principle.

There are certain pointers that must be attended to in treatment. The digestive organs must receive prior attention, as also should the organs of elimination. The spinal areas of the body are represented by the medial aspect of each foot: the big toe being the head, and down its side the cervicals. Attention to these zones would relieve any spinal segment congestions and also would affect the autonomic nervous system. Pay attention to flat feet, as this condition may result in troubles of the colon, such as constipation or a toxic state.

When a therapist locates a tense area, the patient will inform him or her of the pain – it is the crystalline deposits present on a nerve ending which makes it feel as if many pieces of glass are being rubbed into the skin. Actually, the therapist does not massage the feet but literally compresses the area or spot. The aim is to free these crystalline deposits, breaking them up and thus dispersing them, and this relieves any pressure there may have been on the nerve endings.

Working on the feet has a direct influence on the lymphatics of the body, an area that has been neglected by all fields of medicine. It is surprising how deep the reaction of these blocked areas in the feet can be.

Reflexologists, aromatherapists, acupuncturists, osteopaths and chiropractors sometimes find that in their work they can bring relief to people with hearing problems. This is not some empty statement, but can be compared to how, when one throws a stone into the water, there is a rippling effect in ever-increasing circles. I have often seen with frequent air travellers, with divers, or with people who have been in close proximity to an explosion, how the messages of hearing to the brain have become blocked. When the energy flow can be regularised, the sense of hearing is often regained.

It is said that sound is transmitted into three stages. When people become aware of a hearing impairment, or can no longer stand loud noises, apparently causing deafness, they should not forget that any of the above-named therapists can possibly bring relief. Helen Keller said: 'I am just as deaf as I am blind.' The problems of deafness are deeper and more complex, if not more important than those of blindness. Deafness is a much worse misfortune because it means the loss of the most vital stimulus: 'the sound of the voice that brings language', as Fred Astaire described it. It was John Keats who said: 'In the intellectual company of man, if I could live again I should do much more than I have for the deaf. I have found deafness a much greater handicap than blindness.' Perhaps that answers the question with which I started this chapter. Neither deafness nor blindness is a minor problem; therefore always seize a chance of help.

Consider for a moment some of the sayings with which we are all familiar: 'to lend an ear', 'to listen with open ears', 'to give a hearing to' – to quote but a few. Children are often accused of not listening to the advice of their parents, or their teacher. Let me explain that hearing is not only a physical phenomenon, because it is also a function of the emotional body which needs to maintain harmony with other functions in the body.

LASER THERAPY

Paul Nogier, a pioneer of auricular acupuncture, also played a large role in the development of laser treatment. In this field he has shown us how laser treatment applied to some of the acupuncture points in the ear can be very successful for people with hearing problems. A very good friend of mine, Dr Richard Talbot, investigated some very interesting angles of laser treatment and applied his knowledge to the treatment of hearing deficiencies. A new laser therapy method was introduced in the *British Journal of Acupuncture* in 1975; although the article was written some twenty years ago, I still find it interesting today.

The first semi-conductor laser was made in 1963. The main characteristic of laser is the monochromicity. The instrument referred to uses a wavelength of 904 nanometres, to which the skin is transparent. The waves penetrate about 2 cm with a maximum power output of 30 mW and this is sufficient to treat the majority of the acupuncture points in the body. The treatment can be given to ear points either by using the narrow beam width of the laser or with a high degree of accuracy by passing the beam along a plastic rod on to the localised point.

In general, the appeal of laser treatment to the acupuncturist is because so many people still show an aversion to needles. Laser treatment combined with other methods such as reflexology is very successful in the treatment of arthritic and traumatic conditions of the small joints of hands and feet. Other major benefits are the rapid reduction of trauma to tendons, the softening of scar tissue and dispersion of haematomas.

Lasers are a relatively new arrival on the scientific scene. The theory of lasers was first put forward by Professor Albert Einstein as long ago as 1917, but the right type of equipment was not available. In fact, so many uses for the laser had been invented before the equipment could be made that lasers were jokingly called 'the solutions chasing problems'. In the late 1950s the practical possibility of an optical laser was demonstrated by Sehawlow and Iownes. The first ruby laser was produced by Dr Theodore Maiman of the Hughes Aircraft Company in the USA. The heart of this first laser was a cube of man-made ruby. The first semi-conductor laser was made in 1963. It is now possible to make lasers based on solids, gases and liquids.

The reason that lasers were hailed as such an advance is because the special properties of the light which they emit. The word 'laser' is short for light amplification by stimulated emission of radiation. The normal source of light, for example a light bulb, produces radiation which is emitted spontaneously. In a laser the material that is emitting the light is said to be stimulated to radiate. Conditions are more controlled and the light has more attractive properties.

We live in an age of noise. Many parents are at loggerheads with their children because of the loudness of the music they play, but probably this is their way of escaping from the pressures of their young lives. The earth has been called the womb of the solar system and cosmic energy is at work here. Natural energy will create a conductive atmosphere of harmony from negative and positive energies, expressed in a language we can understand and convey to others, if we consider ourselves part of that Creation.

CASE HISTORIES

I will follow here the pattern set in previous chapters by providing some case histories. A gentleman in his early seventies explained to me that he felt his hearing ability had lately become impaired. I immediately realised during my examination that he suffered from a good deal of congestion. This is usually experienced in the chest, but I also found signs of this in his ears and his nose. Sadly, I had to diagnose that his condition had been neglected. I determined that strong measures were called for, and chose a remedy developed by a Dutch biochemist that is based on enzymes. From experience I have great faith in this remedy and know that it is very worth while in the treatment of congestion.

After only three days the first effects become noticeable, in that he began to discharge a great deal of mucus. The patient then happily reported that he heard his ears pop, and his hearing greatly improved. He was so delighted with the outcome of this remedy, that he has vowed to continue using it. The name of this enzyme-based remedy is Enzybios, and it has stood me in good stead with quite a few patients, for many cases of congestion and also when an anti-histamine was required.

Then there was a 28-year-old female patient with tinnitus. In her own words, not only was she driven mad by the noises reverberating around her head, she also suffered unpleasant and inconvenient dizzy spells. which had gradually started to undermine her confidence. She had consulted all the doctors and specialists she could think of, but none of the medication or treatments she was prescribed had brought about an improvement in her condition. I did not underestimate the challenge and started with electro-acupuncture, but the deciding factor in the eventual success was the remedies I prescribed:

- Bioforce *Gingko biloba* (fifteen drops, three times daily)
- Enzymatic therapy's Hexaniacin (one capsule, twice daily, after meals)
- Nature's Best's vitamin B12 (one tablet daily with a meal)

I often hear criticism about the use of vitamin B12, as it is usually maintained that it is only good for blood-forming, but in cases such as this I find that it is very effective. Vitamin B12 is a complex substance containing the mineral cobalt at its centre. Principally, it participates in the rapid regeneration of bone marrow and red blood cells. This vitamin was first isolated from the liver in 1948 and is needed for the synthesis of DNA and for normal metabolism of nerve tissue. Folic acid, iron and vitamin B12 are all referred to as haematinic factors and are vital for the formation of healthy blood cells. Vitamin B12 is also necessary for myelin sheath production in nerve tissue.

My patient used these remedies for some time and, as her blood pressure occasionally showed a tendency to rise, I also prescribed Arterioforce capsules. Arterioforce is a Bioforce remedy with *Crataegus oxyacantha* (hawthorn berry) as its main ingredient. It is frequently prescribed for complaints such as hardening of the arteries and signs of senility, to decrease the effects of arteriosclerosis and to increase the capacity for activity. Depending on the circumstances, it is also considered a useful remedy for itchiness, listlessness, memory loss or impairment, dizziness, slightly elevated blood pressure, difficulty in ability to concentrate, and loss of vitality. The combined treatment had the required effect and, needless to say, my patient was delighted.

Then I want to tell you about a teenager whose symptoms included swollen tonsils, chronic earache, slight deafness and infrequent noises in the head. When I did an iridology test, using Chinese facial diagnosis techniques, I soon discovered a considerable toxic problem. His lymph glands were swollen, so I decided that he was an ideal candidate for a detoxification programme and prescribed Dr Vogel's De-Tox Box. This programme was developed by Dr Vogel and myself many years ago and we often refer to it as the 'Spring Cleansing Course'. I myself follow this programme every spring and every autumn. The programme is designed to cleanse the gall-bladder, liver, kidneys, stomach and lungs. Dietary restrictions are part of this cleansing course and in this young lad's case I also suggested that he should refrain from eating dairy foods. His initial improvement was rapid, after which he gradually returned to his former self.

Then there was a middle-aged lady who was complaining of dizziness. Although she had been receiving treatment from her GP, her dizzy spells continued, and she had also been prescribed *Cocculus* by a homoeopathic practitioner. I have seen some good results with this remedy, but the lady in question had not benefited from using it. When I checked her blood pressure it was somewhat higher than I would have liked to see, but my main concern was her poor circulation. I decided to prescribe *Viscum album* (three times a day, ten drops before meals) and also *Gingko biloba* (three times daily, fifteen drops after meals). The prescribed treatment was completed by the homoeopathic remedy *Tabacum* D4. I asked her to replace her usual coffee with a coffee substitute from Bioforce, called Bambu, which contains no caffeine. As a salt replacement I suggested Herbamare, Dr Vogel's seasoning salt. Herbamare is prepared with fresh, organically grown herbs. The fresh herbs are combined with natural sea salt and allowed to steep for six to eight weeks before the moisture is removed by a special vacuum process at low temperature. I agree with Dr Vogel, who always maintained that this would greatly benefit people with blood pressure problems. My patient wrote to me some time later to express her gratitude.

Another male patient, aged thirty-two, had catarrhal deafness and, as he was a postman, this complaint frequently recurred according to the weather conditions. I started with dietary advice, and also suggested a brief fast, during which period he would take no solids but fruit and vegetable juices only, e.g. beetroot and carrot juice. Furthermore, I gave him osteopathic treatment. I used a method I had learned years ago in America, a method that seems to be no longer in fashion, yet I still occasionally employ it because of its effectiveness in certain circumstances. For this treatment it is necessary to insert the fingers into the mouth where slight manipulation is practised until the Eustachian tube opens up. This proved an excellent therapy for this gentleman's condition. I also prescribed Echinaforce (twenty drops, three times a day) and some vitamin supplements such as Imuno Strength (one tablet, twice daily).

An elderly lady consulted me because she had always enjoyed exceptionally good hearing, but had recently noticed a rapid deterioration. I could not detect any unusual signs of catarrh, but when questioned she told me that she worked in a noisy area. I have already mentioned earlier that in today's environment our five senses are being constantly stressed and good care should be taken. In the case of this lady, although there was no catarrhal deafness, she had restricted movement in her neck. This indicated that she would likely benefit from spinal manipulation and I concentrated on the first three cervical vertebrae, with very good results.

The case of a five-year-old child was very unusual. This child had badly impaired hearing, on one side only, while she also frequently complained of earache on that same side. On thorough examination I discovered a small object lodged in the ear. Imagine our surprise when I discovered that the foreign object was a green pea. At some time the little girl, in a playful mood, presumably lacking interest in her food, must have stuffed a pea in her ear. When I made this discovery the pea had already started sprouting and it needed great care and deftness to remove it. I disinfected the child's ear and then advised the mother to take the child to an ENT specialist, and fortunately it was later confirmed that no permanent harm had been done.

A 37-year-old employee at the local airport consulted me because of a condition that seemed to be developing into a semi-permanent earache and I diagnosed a middle ear infection. She had had some very extensive antibiotic treatment, but unfortunately the earache continued to recur. I prescribed Echinaforce (twenty drops before meals, twice daily) and *Plantago* (twice daily, twenty drops after meals). I also suggested that before going to sleep she should place a piece of cotton-wool sprinkled with no more than five drops of *Plantago* into the ear. Furthermore, she should take twice a day a Phytobiotic capsule from Enzymatic Therapy. Within no time at all we had managed to reverse the condition.

We should bear in mind that there is always hope. If one thing fails, never give up, but try something else. There is nearly always a solution, and we must never give up. Nature is our very best friend and there are so many useful remedies that have proven their worth, where stronger orthodox medical treatment has failed.

5

Vision

It came as quite a shock to me some years ago when an ophthalmologist warned me that I should realise that one day I might be blind. Initially I was sceptical because I have always had good eyes, but then I remembered that in later life my grandmother had lost her eyesight, and my mother's eyesight had also deteriorated very badly in her latter years. What was a definite weakness in the family might eventually take its toll on me. Immediately upon this realisation I determined that action was called for and decided to look for every possible way to avoid following in my family's footsteps.

Possibly as the result of this warning, I must admit that I have a great interest in people with visual impairment. I return to the opening question of the previous chapter, about what would be worse: being deaf or being blind. Either problem is certainly sufficiently serious to try everything possible to avoid reaching that stage.

There are many ways in which we can help ourselves and there is no doubt that because of today's technology, and I am thinking specifically about word processors, computers and televisions, the demands on our eyesight are certainly greater than in years gone by. The many people with visual impairment I have treated over the years and who have been successful in retaining or regaining their eyesight, are those who have followed the advice with enthusiasm.

The eyes are a truly wonderful feat of design. They are orbs with an average diameter of 2 to 2.5 cm, and they can move by using no more than six little muscles. The eyes are of such miraculous design that they can bend light rays and bring them into focus on the retina. Without any conscious thought or intention the eye can focus on any object by contracting the tiny circular muscles around the lens, making the lens fatter, and when focusing on a more distant object, the radial muscles contract to allow us to see it more clearly. All the transparent elements of the eye – the conjunctiva, the cornea and the fluid – contribute to the power we have in the eyes. We soon realise how marvellous the design of the eye is, if we think that at either end of the eye is a minuscule fountain that ensures that anything that comes into the eye will be immediately flushed away.

The eyeball consists of three distinct layers of tissue: a tough outer layer called the sclera; the choroid layer, which is supplied with tiny blood vessels and pigmented to stop light escaping through the back of the eye; and the light-sensitive retina. The retina is easily damaged and we have to be very careful when there is pressure behind the eye or a possible leakage of blood.

In dim light 125 million receptors around the eye and retina see shapes in black, light and grey. In bright light stimulation of seven million receptors behind the central area of the retina takes place. The light-sensitive pigment inside these, called rhodopsin, which is replaced during sleep, requires nourishment. There is a standing joke that a rabbit does not need glasses because it eats a lot of carrots. This root vegetable is a good provider of vitamin A, and this is a vitamin that provides nourishment to the eyes.

The pigmented muscular iris controls the amount of light reaching the retina and the conjuctiva, which is a continuation of the epidermis; it is constantly cleared by the tear glands, and sometimes needs assistance. If there is a blockage in the tear duct it needs immediate attention. Unfortunately, too many people know what it is like to lose their vision, yet many more are fortunate in that if they take the usual care, they will never have to experience such loss. Think of the biblical quotation, 'Where there is no vision, the people perish' (Proverbs 29:18). It is therefore extremely important to take good care of this gift.

In his book *Better Sight Without Glasses* Harry Benjamin writes in detail about defective vision, and explains how this can sometimes be overcome by dietary measures, exercises and relieving stress. He states that we need not look at the eye itself for the causes of eye disease, but that we should examine the entire body. Eyes, the mirrors of the body, can reveal many problems which may remain hidden elsewhere within. Iridology is a science that can help us to reveal the source of many hidden problems.

The sensors of the eye are located immediately behind them and if we know what to look for they can serve as alarm signals. If we take heed of their message we can forestall major health problems. In the first instance, excessive brain work and tension can place a tremendous strain on our eyes, as does artificial light, especially neon light. The same applies to VDUs (visual display units), i.e. the screens used for word processors, computers and television. In my experience I have seen a major difference when I treat people who live in the country and work on the land. If we were to reduce our reliance on some of the methods that modern technology has provided, I am sure that our eyesight would benefit. Before the advent of television people used to go out for a stroll in the evening. This is what they used to call their constitutional, and there is no doubt that their eyesight benefited. Eyes are exposed to excessive strain due to artificial light, year after year, and this will indeed take its toll, and we become increasingly out of tune with Nature.

We also know that the pineal glands needs cosmic light. Just think what happens to flowers and plants when they have to do without natural light: they wither and die. This also applies to the human body. It will wither if it does not get sufficient fresh air and oxygen. I remember at one stage Dr Vogel became very worried about excessive watering from his tear ducts. One evening after a lecture he told me that his eyes were telling him that the strain was becoming too great, because we were spending too much time indoors, on brightly lit stages. Bacteria, dust and other foreign particles are usually washed away by tears, but during our lecture tours the conditions were such that our tear ducts became impaired, and the necessary watering of the eyes was reduced. The lachrimal glands had become inflamed. I remember being surprised at the way he set about repairing or minimising the damage: because he used warm milk and mallow leaf water, with one or two drops of Echinaforce to bathe the eyes at night, and this helped him greatly. I still remember that he used to expound his theory on how eyes were a miracle and that we owed it to ourselves to safeguard them in whatever way possible.

One of my grandchildren was born prematurely and her eyes are like an open book. Looking into her eyes gives the impression that you can see right into her. Because the eyes are the mirrors of the soul it is easy to imagine that we can see what she thinks, and that is a feeling that I experience, especially with young animals and young children. The eye can look friendly, and it can look angry. It can be activated and it can be blind. Often we wonder why we sometimes take an immediate like or dislike to someone. Think of the expression that love is blind, and one realises how much truth there is in that saying. We often see this with myopic people, who look at people in a different manner, and it seems as if they are capable of seeing only one thing, or one person, at a time. There is no distraction in what is happening around them, because they appear to be concentrating on just that one image. This reminds me of the story of the apostle Paul who on his way to Damascus intended to kill the first Christians who followed in the ways of Christ. His eyes were covered with his own thoughts and he was locked in his own opinions, when God opened his eyes to see what he was doing. When his eyes were uncovered he was blind, and after that God removed the scales from his eyes and showed him a vision and that sudden insight allowed him to become one of the greatest people on earth.

Sometimes we can see the meaning behind the symptoms and this is often the case with conjunctivitis, which is usually brought on by stress or conflict, either at home or at work. Conjunctivitis is often associated psychologically with issues we do not want to think about or, conversely, are not being able to see beyond. To have clear vision is important, because all too often there are instances when at a later stage we must admit that we were 'slain with blindness'. However, think of the things we want to see in a realistic light. When we come to a deeper understanding of our inner selves, we are able to develop a knowledge of our three bodies: the mental, physical and emotional bodies. Emotionally we may come to recognise that we are sometimes slain with blindness because we refuse to face up to things.

Think of the expression that 'it is all in the eye of the beholder'. If we look at ourselves in the mirror, and make the effort to look into our own eyes, we must wonder what affects our bodies mentally, physically and emotionally. We should then ask ourselves whether the mind, body and soul are in harmony.

Sometimes very little is required to regain harmony. A female patient at my clinic had very troubled vision. Some of this was indeed self-inflicted, but some of it was due to her personality. She was an extremely conscientious person; she took personal responsibility for everything that came across her path, and generally worried about everything. However, during her check-up I recognised a miasma. A miasma is a left-over from a previous inflammation, virus or infection, that can actually be present from previous generations. In this lady's case I found a miasma of tuberculosis, for which I prescribed a homoeopathic nosode of Tuberculinum. She soon felt better and at the same time her vision improved greatly. As well as the homoeopathic nosode, I also prescribed some exercises, and the change in her condition was surprising.

Our eyes are a miracle, as vision is a miracle. The eyes are organs of light as well as of sight. The eyes rotate around three axes: vertical, horizontal and oblique.

Next to life itself, sight is man's most precious possession. In spite of this fact we make very little effort to conserve our vision. Vision is not a simple process but a somewhat complex one – although normal vision appears easy and natural.

The functions of the eyes are well co-ordinated, and usually bad habits of use, misuse and abuse are the cause of almost all strain and eye troubles. Strain will cause interference with the blood, lymph and nerve supply, and we should remember that these are the lifelines of all tissue. Weak eyes are often found in unhealthy bodies and disturbed vision is not of a refractive nature, although it is often treated as such.

Healthy eyes depend on perfect nutrition, drainage and nerve supply. A greater appreciation of vision is not necessary, but a great knowledge of eye care is. The care and conservation of vision begins at home, not in the schoolroom or the doctor's surgery. The eye is a very delicate precision-constructed piece of nervous mechanism, and it must have free circulation of blood, lymph and nerve currents, as well as rest, otherwise there will be visual dysfunction.

Natural treatment aims to correct bad habits by training and treatment. Often it is necessary to treat some pathological condition before visual training can start. Revitalising the nervous elements and correcting bad habits by natural methods can take the form of hydrotherapy, massage, exercise and diet supplemented by electrotherapy, eye training and chiropractic adjustment.

The conservation of vision does not begin by wearing glasses to protect your eyes. Glasses are only a form of support; they do not cure eye-strain or correct the condition that causes eye-strain. This applies to young adults and middle-aged people as well as to children. Children should be watched especially carefully, as weak eyes can often follow children's diseases. Convalescence after sickness is a critical time. Strong light should be avoided and only limited reading and television should be allowed. Late hours and unnecessary excitement should be avoided, while plenty of rest – possibly including an afternoon nap – is to be encouraged. Attention to all these factors can improve weak and defective vision.

There are several laws of life that will also affect the eyes. These are as follows:

1. Oxidation – the keystone of health. Life is in the blood. Oxygen is the bridge between life and death; between health and disease.
2. Elimination – removal of waste. The accumulation of waste in the

body with its toxic by-products will kill you in twenty-four hours.
3. Nutrition – the building and repair of the body. The energy to function is maintained by the use of oxygen in the tissues.
4. Motion – or work. The vibration, expansion and contraction of cells, muscles and tissues.
5. Relaxation – rest. The least expenditure of energy while still keeping the body functioning.

The blood is purified by oxygen in the lungs. All people who are suffering from ill health lack blood oxygen. Bacteria cannot live in pure oxygen or pure blood. If the respiratory tract is obstructed, oxygen starvation results, leading not only to disease of the open cavities in the nose, throat and ears, but also in the closed cavities elsewhere in the body.

The five most important functions of oxygen are as follows:

1. It has combustible units of gas that give off heat. These units of heat make soluble nutritional elements fit for absorption by the body.
2. Vapour or water that keeps the gas in solution has a dissolving power greater than any other element entering the body. This moisture combined with heat melts secretions and renders them liquid for elimination.
3. Oxygen attracts iron to the body. This is one of the essential elements for stamina and virility.
4. Oxygen maintains cell rate virility.
5. Oxygen is an aid to the sinuses for balance of the body and resonance of the voice.

Oxidation is life. You can be paralysed and live, but you cannot live without oxygen no matter how many adjustments you make. The process of exchange of carbon dioxide for oxygen is continuous, ending only at death. The rate of exchange may be fast or slow.

EXERCISES
Some useful exercises for eye muscle problems, visual defects and headaches follow below. At this point I will add that any condition related to the eyes will benefit from the use of vitamin A, of which

carrots are a good provider. However, great benefit can also be had from eating 2 oz of sunflower seeds daily, as they are also rich in vitamin A.

Some simple things we can do to help our eyes

1. Holding the fingers before the nose, spread and wiggle the fingers.
2. Look at a large clock, follow the figures around the clock and reverse the procedure. Then do it with the eyes closed as well.
3. Place the fingers of either hand at the tip of the nose, then extend to arm's length and follow the movement with the eyes, before returning the hand to the eyes. Reverse the action.
4. Face the sun and then, through closed eyelids, look at the sun. Then place the fingers before the eyes and slowly open the fingers, like a lattice work and gaze at the sun through it, opening and closing the eyelids as well as the fingers. Open and flutter the eyelids.
5. Write imaginary words with the tip of the nose. This is difficult but is beneficial and speedy results can be obtained.
6. Place a card in front of the face at the nose. Block out the central vision and use the peripheral vision. This makes the peripheral muscles work. In a car do the same (if not driving) and note the passing telegraph poles. Hold the card thus till the eyes tingle, which means that they are tired.
7. Exercise the eyes every morning, noon and night, for between two and five minutes. Rotate the eyes in an imaginary circle as large as possible, first to the left, then to the right – ten times each way.
8. Roll the eyes as high as possible, as if attempting to look into the brain, then down as if trying to look into the roof of the mouth – ten times. Look to the left side without turning the head – as far as possible; then to the right. Ten times in each direction.
9. Place the fingers over the optical nerves, just above the temples, and massage with a revolving motion over the ear and down the neck to relax the nerves.
10. Recharge the phosphorus with the ultra-violet rays of the morning sun. Watch the sun come up in the morning and do not wear your glasses while exercising or watching the sun rise.
11. Remove the glasses gradually, for five or ten minutes at a time. Do not expect to remove them at once for good. Soon the eyes will become

sufficiently strong to discard them all together.

12. Always place the light behind you or to the side when reading. When the source of light is in front of you, the beams fall on the work and are reflected into the eyes directly. This causes severe strain, and with poor food and lack of exercise would have detrimental effects.

Human beings – as opposed to some animals – usually look straight ahead and so we lose our peripheral vision. Also, we do not roll our eyes in their sockets.

Dr Allan once gave me a leaflet which he in turn had been given by Dr Hollie, who specialised in the study of the eyes. Dr Hollie wrote that eyes are very sensitive and the most precious part of the body.

Ask yourself how much your eyes are worth. Guard them as you would your most precious possession. Glasses do not cure eyes that are weak, and as the eyesight deteriorates, glasses must be exchanged for stronger lenses. Anyone who can still see, can have good eyesight, providing there has been no external injury.

The eyes are just as much part of the body as the hands and feet, and therefore need a certain amount of exercise. The physical parts of the eyes are built principally from sulphur and phosphorus. The part that gives us the light in our eyes is built from the ultra-violet rays of the morning sun. Window glass and the glass from which eye glasses are made eliminate these ultra-violet rays.

A further exercise when the eyes and sinuses are involved is a method which activates an energy impulse to release the sinus areas. This, however, requires a practitioner as it cannot be practised alone. The feet must be tested for any soreness under each toe except the big toe, because if the eyes or the sinus areas are involved, there will often be tenderness.

The patient must lie on his back, while the therapist stands on the right side. Begin by touching the underneath of the patient's right toes with the fingers of the right hand and place the right thumb on the bottom of the big toe. The tips of the left-hand fingers then make contact with the patient's right-hand fingers.

Ask the patient to take six deep breaths slowly whilst doing the same yourself.

There is one more movement sequence that is essential: whilst breathing in, direct the patient to move his and your fingers to the shoulder area. On breathing out move down toward the right hip. Then touch the patient's left toes (underneath) with your left hand, and the patient's fingers with your right hand.

The same breathing process is repeated – up to the left shoulder on inhalation and down to the left hip on exhalation. Usually, after the six breathing cycles, the tender areas under the toes will have gone.

Usually after this energy cycle the patient will feel lightheaded as if floating on air. Sinus relief will also be greatly appreciated.

Exercises are of great help for the retina which consists of nerve tissue – in a developing unborn baby it is actually part of the brain itself. It may surprise you to learn that there are more than 130 million sight-receiving cells located in the retina which connect with the sight centre of the brain. This is one of the reasons why the eye is so sensitive. I often advise people who suffer from tired eyes to carefully place a finger of the left hand on each eye with the lids closed. Clasp the lids with the right hand and very gently make them vibrate. This is a most energising and relaxing treatment for the eye and can be done without fear of harming it. Vibration of the eye towards the nose is also relaxing.

I often advise people to use the Benjamin method. Dr Benjamin's book *Perfect Sight Without Glasses* describes from personal experience the effects his method can have on normal, affected and poor sight. With the advice in his book Dr Benjamin has been able to help many people with visual problems. He has often applied the Alexander technique, which is a good balancing technique that I have also suggested to many of my patients. Dr Benjamin's technique was developed largely by his own experiments, but he has complemented this with some sections of the Alexander technique. He also advised using Flower Remedies; like me, he is a great advocate of Emergency Essence, which can help to correct many problems if taken as soon as the need presents itself.

TREATING DRY EYES

Although there are many more eye disorders, in recent years the incidence of dry eyes appears to be increasing. Dry eye disorders are a complex group of diseases that can be characterised by:

1. a localised water deficiency in the tear ducts
2. a mucin deficiency
3. a combination of the above

Despite the diversity of underlying causes, the changes in the conjunctiva of the eye are similar in all cases, i.e. loss of goblet cells (mucin-producing cells), abnormal enlargement of non-goblet epithelial cells, and an increase of cellular layers and keratin deposition, stratification and keratinisation.

Other than topical vitamin A therapy, all other non-surgical therapies for dry eyes, such as the frequent application of artificial tears, lubricants or slow-releasing polymers, and the therapeutic use of soft contact lenses, are not directed toward reversing the underlying process, but rather toward alleviating the symptoms.

The hypothesis that a localised vitamin A deficiency in the lining of the outer eye may be responsible for dry eyes, considering vitamin A's vital role in epithelial tissue, seems obvious. Clinical studies featuring a commercial vitamin A eye-drop formula (Viva-Drops from Vision Pharmaceuticals) have yielded impressive clinical results in the treatment of dry eyes. Unlike other dry eye preparations, however, the underlying cellular changes causing the dry eyes are reversed by topical vitamin A.

NUTRITION

At the risk of repeating myself, I must emphasise again that prevention is always better than cure – which is one of the main reasons I decided to write this book. I stress again that the five senses are very much affected in today's society. My great friend Carolyn Gazella recently wrote an article on the eyes, in which she mentioned the old saying: 'You don't know what you've got, until it's gone.' If ever this was true, it applies to our sight. We take our sight very much for granted and do so little to protect it, and yet, when our sight is diminishing, we are surprised.

Few people recognise how important nutrition is for the eyes. The *Nutrition Research Newsletter* reported on a 1993 study carried out in Canada which found that people who did not take vitamin E were two and a half times more likely to develop cataracts. The risk for those who did not take vitamin C was four times higher. A 1994 study conducted at the Harvard Medical School showed that antioxidants can reduce the risk of developing macula degeneration by half. Yet another study conducted by the US Department of Agriculture and Human Research Center on Ageing at Tufts University discovered that low betacarotene levels were associated with an increased risk of a certain type of cataract, while low vitamin C levels were associated with an increased risk for still another type of cataract. Bioflavonoids are also important and Professor David Newsome, clinical professor of ophthalmology at Tulane University School of Medicine, has stated that there is a similar link with macula degeneration in cataracts.

In addition to people who have a family history of sight defects, it is estimated that each year some 15,000–30,000 diabetics and people taking prescription drugs lose their sight. In adults between the ages of twenty-five and seventy-four, diabetes accounts for the majority of cases. It is said that there are more than two million people with glaucoma in the USA. Glaucoma is a disease of the eye marked by increased pressure in the eyeball as the result of an imbalance. It can lead to all kinds of problems, ranging from pain to nausea and chronic loss of peripheral vision, resulting in tunnel vision, conjunctivitis and gradual loss of sight. In such cases it is wise to take extra vitamin C, and often bilberry extract is prescribed. With cataracts, the use of amino acids is recommended in combination with other vitamins: eyebright, chamomile, fennel, vitamin C and zinc are all useful supplements. More details on this subject can be found in the case histories.

The eye is one of the most intricate organs and works like a sophisticated camera, taking millions of pictures each day. Vision takes place when light rays are focused on the small area at the centre of the retina, but we also have to bear in mind the *mental* side of seeing. The brain interprets the meaning of the impulses that are sent from the retina. Clear vision is the result if we can react quickly to the visual impulses of the retina and for this it is important to learn to relax our mind as well as our eyes.

Trying to improve memory and visualisation can be achieved by improved muscle control – and this book contains much advice on this subject, approached from various angles. Apart from exercises there are a number of treatment methods that can be useful in improving our precious eyesight.

LIGHT AND COLOUR THERAPIES

The most important factor for our eyesight is light. The first step in Creation was the birth of light out of darkness, and we are all familiar with the gratitude and relief we experience when we glimpse the first ray of light after having been in darkness for any length of time. Light is not only the medicine of the future, it is also the miracle of Creation. I have read with great interest the latest book by Steven Hawking, the well-known Oxford scientist. He writes about his vision of where and how Creation began, but I doubt if any of us will ever know for sure. Many great scientists have given us their personal views, but as it is impossible to behold eternity, so it is with Creation. Time that is created out of eternity is measured for us to exist in our daily life. I have lasting memories of a conversation with my uncle, who held a managerial position in one of the most advanced mental hospitals in the Netherlands. He maintained that there were too many patients who had tried to grasp what it all means, and that was their reason for being hospitalised.

The future of medicine is in energy – and light is one of the most important aspects of energy. Light is capable of travelling faster than any other known phenomenon and it is barely possible to understand its significance. As eyes depend on light, vision will become clearer, and with the combined exercise of light and colour we may be able to achieve an improvement in our eyesight, resulting in being able to cope with weaker lenses in our spectacles.

Focusing on a single item is not always the answer. Visualisation therapy can be remarkably successful and it is possible to train oneself by visualising or concentrating with single-mindedness on improving one's eyesight. I was greatly interested to read an excellent book, *Light – Medicine of the Future*, by Jacob Lieberman. In this book I read about a certain Harry Riley Spittler who, in 1919, performed an intriguing experiment on young rabbits. He took a number of baby rabbits and placed them in individual cages, where he gave them the same amounts of food and water, and exactly the same treatment, except that he varied their exposure to light. Some rabbits had yellow light in their cages, others blue or white. Although the experiment was designed to last for a period of two years, within three months he became aware of some interesting changes. Some of the rabbits developed at a fast rate, while others seemed to stagnate. Some rabbits had full and healthy coats, and other suffered hair loss. Anxiety and depression was noticeable among some of the rabbits. He carefully recorded any changes in the condition of these rabbits and his conclusion was that underlying vision problems were causing imbalances in the autonomic nervous system and the endocrine system. He felt that the light received through the eyes directly affected these systems. He continued with his training and applied his findings to visual as well as physical problems. In 1933 he formed a group called the College of Symptonic Optometry.

In his book Jacob Lieberman also describes how he treated his mother who had lost her eyesight. He experimented with several different colours, but because she had optic neuritis he used the colour blue-green. The first breakthrough came when, after twenty days of treatment, his mother was able to read several letters from a distance of approximately twenty feet. This was an encouraging and eye-opening experience for Jacob Lieberman. He compares the body to a living photocell, stimulated and regulated by light entering the eyes – the windows of our soul. He places emphasis on the significance of nutrition and malnutrition and mentions a number of conditions that can lead to eye trouble.

Before the beginning of time darkness reigned on earth. Time was the first and most essential thing and God commanded: 'Let there be light'. In this way He created time, being the difference between light and darkness and the tools capable of reacting to light, in other words, time became the eyes. The eye transmits messages to the hypothalamus and there is a close connection between the hypothalamus and the pineal gland. It is this connection that is often affected in patients suffering from myalgic encephalomyelitis (ME) or post-viral fatigue syndrome. It is frequently noticed with such patients that the eyes seem heavy.

Is it true that blue light can help arthritis and that red light is beneficial to migraine sufferers? Purple light is claimed to be dangerous to individuals with cancer and leukaemia. There is little doubt that light in its full spectrum of colour has an influence on our health. It is with the balance of light that God has created that gives us such a powerful tool for healing. We know the power of sunlight and how it provides us with vitamins. We also know the power of darkness. In this great concept of light we cannot fail to acknowledge the value of light and colour.

The great pioneering work of Dr John Pott in the United States, with whom I have corresponded for many years, has shown me how light can work. In one particular case I found three children with leukaemia in one classroom, and I called on him for advice. Could it be that colour played a role here? He asked me to report on the entire environment of these children, at home and at school, paying special attention to the colours that were prevalent in their daily lives. When I reported the colour scheme in the classroom, he remarked about the unfortunate disharmony of colour to which these children were exposed during a major part of their day, and that these would be influential in their particular illness.

Colour is a life force. Dr Hazel Parcells, whom I have known and admired for many years, was over one hundred years old when she died. She viewed colour as 'the life force in the human body', and she also referred to herself as the best 'kitchen chemist', as she knew how to combine a healthy nutritional diet with light and colour treatment. Her successes were usually very impressive and sometimes beyond belief.

In the case of strong lighting, or very powerful sunlight, we are subjected to a state of disharmony. Unfortunately, skin cancer has become more and more prevalent in recent years. Harmony in the seven layers of light receptors in the retina is as important as it is in the seven colours of the rainbow. The lack of harmony can result in significant health problems. Albert Einstein remarked that such problems 'could not be solved on the same level of thinking as where and when we created them'.

Light and colour are only the tip of the iceberg. There is an enormous field of energy that has not yet been fully explored or understood. It is indeed important to work with light and this is often confirmed during acupuncture treatment sessions. I often combine this method with light or colour therapy and I always make sure that the colours are well balanced. Also with aromatherapy treatment it is important to use colours that are in harmony. Ancient healers showed an inherent understanding of the requirement of harmony in light and colours, and this is borne out in their rituals as well as in their religions. Dr Dinshah P. Ghadiali, who lived from 1873 to 1966, was the originator of spectrochrome therapy and he has left behind a wealth of knowledge about what can be done with light and colour, and how spectrochrome colour can be applied for the benefit of health.

Going back several decades to the war years, a whole generation spent their formative years in rooms where the windows were covered by black paper, or in underground shelters, to safeguard themselves against the ravages of bombardments. Everything appeared black – physically, mentally and emotionally – and death and destruction reigned. As a young boy I also was forced to experience such deprivation.

I was fairly young when I discovered colour. When I was in total darkness I started to visualise things in colour and realised that we were surrounded by colour. Every now and then I spent some time with an elderly gentleman who showed me a three-dimensional instrument and some photographs, and he told me about coloured lights he had used. It made a great impression on me during those dark times.

Every time I visit Arnhem in the Netherlands I make a point of driving past a very special place. I used to sit in a house there with this old gentleman while he opened up a whole new world with his viewer. This house was bombed during the Second World War, just one hour after I had been sitting there. I lived in this house with my mother, where she cared for some elderly people and refugees. It was thanks to my mother's intuition that we were not still in the house when it was bombed and flattened. This is why I make a point of reliving my memory.

I have many memories such as these, because it was in those dark days that I learnt to appreciate and value life. My elderly friend opened a world of colour to me and I regarded him with the same appreciation as the monk I met at the monastery which was close to the house where I lived. This monastery had one of the finest herb gardens I have ever seen. My old friend, the monk, had lost most of his sight, but on his knees he showed me herbs and plants of which he knew the value with an unerring instinct. I spent hours and hours with the monk, who happily imparted his knowledge to me, and even though quite a lot of it must have gone over my head, it has left an everlasting impression. In the hours that I was forced to spend in darkness during the bombardments, I digested his information and visualised light and colours. These two elderly friends of mine taught me at an early age about the love of God who created life and light and it was in those days that the desire was born in me to help mankind. This desire has never left me.

A very dear friend of mine, Dr Hans Moolenburgh, says that we are only the pen that is being guided by God. Ever since our student days we have had long debates about every subject imaginable, consequentially always returning to the value of life and the tools that are provided by Nature to safeguard this.

When I was still young I already became aware that I associated certain people with specific colours. When I matured I read all I could about what was scientifically proven about the use of colour therapy and how harmony could be brought into colour. I was so engrossed with this particular aspect that I became blind to colour itself, and it took a long time before I regained my vision in this respect.

Later in life I gained much insight from Dr Leonid Gissen, who had assisted Mr Kirlian, who discovered Kirlian photography. Mr Kirlian developed a method that scientifically proves that we are surrounded by colour and that colour can be seen as an outflowing aura from the body. Kirlian photography provides us with evidence that the physical body is a condensation of energy. Harmony, or lack of harmony, in the mind or body produces many observed effects, one of which is a change in the 'field' around the body. This field, which seems to be partly electromagnetic in nature, has been observed to change its form and shape during, and sometimes prior to, the onset of medical and psychological conditions. The hands and the feet, being rich in nervous tissue and acupuncture meridian terminal points, give an accurate picture of this field. When the charged plate of the Kirlian apparatus – with its own regular field – is placed in close proximity to the hands or feet, interference patterns are produced. These are recorded on photographic paper and provide the basis for diagnosis.

Apart from investigating the life energy of plants, food, seeds, etc., Kirlian photography has a dual purpose:

1. To assist in the process of familiarisation and diagnosis when the patient is seen for the first time.
2. To observe the effects of a treatment or therapy.

It is of particular relevance when the patient presents unclear or ambiguous symptoms or does not respond to treatment over a period of time. Specifically, the method can highlight the following features:

- the level of energy patterns of degeneration
- the balance between the two sides of the body (yin and yang)
- the nature and extent of any emotional problems
- the level of physical tension
- the extent of psychological withdrawal
- the general stability of personality
- organic imbalance (correlating with reflexology and acupuncture)
- the degree of a patient's resistance to treatment
- the overall condition of the spine and associated weaknesses

I know that colour can play a major role in people's health. Whenever I notice a disharmony in the outflowing energy aura, this should be restored through harmony – just as in the seven colours of the rainbow. The importance of harmony was continuously in my mind when I composed the flower essences which went on to become such a tremendous success, because I even strived for harmony in the choice of colours of the flowers I used.

People sometimes react with scepticism when I stress the importance of colour harmony, but I am absolutely convinced of its value because we cannot survive without light, and in the spectrum of pure light there exists all the colours of the rainbow; these only become visible to our maladjusted eyes when refracted through a spectral prism, such as raindrops which result in the mysterious rainbow. Without light and colour we would wither emotionally, physically and mentally. There would be no photosynthesis which results in the green colouring called chlorophyll in the leaves of trees and plants, and no oxygen which we need to breathe and circulate our life force. Colours travel through the air as light waves of vibration, which can be measured rather like sound waves are measured in megahertz or nanometres, which we are all familiar with. We have heard of infra-red and ultra-violet rays, and just as we have accepted infra-red and ultra-violet lamps, we must accept the importance of colour. It makes sense that we will be able to calm a turbulent or red situation with a lighter and therefore soothing colour. Turquoise is the complementary colour to red and suggests to us the sea gently rolling onto the shore. If you know what to look for it is easy to understand how much colour influences our lives.

Light and colour are two very important tools for helping people. Their importance lies in the combinations we use and how we apply them in treatment. With the several disciplines we use I often see that their use reinforces the treatment positively. The seven colours in the spectrum are red, orange, yellow, green, blue, indigo and violet, and every one of these colours has an influence on one of the seven endocrine glands.

I spoke the other day with my great friend, Soozi Holbeche, who has been in practice for many years and she maintains that life, love and light are of the utmost importance and that using the right colours to balance these is a major challenge. In the several books she has written she has done much to encourage the understanding of her principles. Even the colours of vibrations are important. Isaac Newton said that when one atom moves, the universe is shaken. Many things can change life on earth and much of it depends on light and colour, if only they are used in the right direction.

It is interesting to contemplate how and why certain colours appeal to certain individuals and personalities. Colour can be used very effectively to express certain personality traits and can also be an equally effective indicator of a person's mental state. For every individual it is important that colour is used in order to bring out certain aspects of their personality. In my book *Menstrual and Pre-Menstrual Tension* I have explained how women who are prone to this complaint can help themselves by changing the colour of the clothes they wear during the week prior to menstruation. Colour therapy harnesses the images of light and the colours of the spectrum. It is an electromagnetic spectrum with a vibrational frequency that cannot be measured. It is of greater importance than is generally realised.

I was pleased to read that in times past religious people used to meditate on colour: blue for relaxation and peace, green for balance and cleansing, violet for dignity and self-respect, and red for love.

The aura of the five senses is related to the five elements: sight is connected with fire, sound is connected with air, taste with the element of water and smell is connected to earth. Touch is of course connected to energy.

During a recent visit to the United States I found a marvellous book written by Theo Gimble, *The Colour Therapy Workbook*. Some of the material in this book was very interesting and one of the phrases he used stuck in my mind: 'Darkness is followed by light; darkness equals light and light follows darkness.' The author suggests that colour is an indicator of health, and described a simple exercise to prove the merits of colour. He suggested choosing a bright and sunny day to conduct the following experiment. Retire to a dark room with the door closed and the windows covered by black paper or cloth. When you have become used to the deep blackness, cut a hole in the paper or cloth, no larger than the palm of the hand. Cover this hole with one of the hands and very soon a small orange light will become noticeable when looking at the hand that is covering the hole. He says that this is actually the complementary colour to the daylight blue of the early afternoon and compares it with a scriptural statement found in John 1:5 that 'the light shineth in darkness and the darkness comprehended it not.'

Ancient philosophers and physicians used colours to represent illness and disease – and just think how the various associations we ascribe to colours are borne out in our language:

- seeing red
- feeling blue
- giving the green light
- going red in the face
- turning green with envy
- the blackness of despair

I remember a young MS patient with very spastic limb movements. When I used colour therapy as part of her treatment she soon became very much calmer. During my time in China I was taught to look, listen and feel. In this process of diagnosing I instinctively apply colours. I see the body as a field of energy: I ask myself during diagnosis where the energy disturbance can be found and how it can be harmonised. The outgoing aura of energy can reveal a great deal of what is going on inside.

By definition, colour is a sensation and the result of stimulation of the retina of light waves of certain lengths. In 1666 Isaac Newton, who formulated the law of gravity, developed the first valuable theory of colour. He stated that sunlight through a prism established the seven basic colours in the spectrum, and these colours are still the same today.

A short time ago Dr Gissen showed me an aura photograph of the brain of a patient. We could not fail to notice the strong colours and we both immediately interpreted the disharmony in the colours as being descriptive of the patient's problems.

Although the diagnostic interpretation or definition of colour therapists may differ slightly, the stimulation transmitted by glands are as follows:

orange: thyroid, memory
lemon: pancreas, thymus

green:	pituitary
blue;	pineal
indigo:	parathyroids
violet:	spleen
magenta:	suprarenals, prostate
scarlet:	testicles, ovaries

Colour also has a tremendous influence on food, and by overcooking food its vital colour is often impaired. When using a microwave not only is the energy of food affected, but also the colour. I recently read the following interesting article written by Edwin D. Babbitt:

> Light being an actual substance moving with peculiar styles of vibrations according to the particular colours which compose it, and at a rate of nearly 186,000 miles a second, it is easy to see that it must have great power, and that the substances receiving it must partake of this power. The fact that the entire world, mineral, vegetable and animal, is ever being transformed into new and beautiful growth, forms and colours under its magic touch, shows its almost omnific power.
>
> Reichenbach (another colour researcher) let water stand in sunlight for five minutes, then a highly sensitive assistant, on drinking it without knowing what was done, immediately said that it was magnetised. It produced a peculiar pepper-like burning on her tongue, palate and throat, down to the stomach, at every point arousing spasmodic symptoms.
>
> Water which stood in the sun twenty minutes was found to be as strongly magnetic as if it had been charged with a nine-layered magnet. Another doctor who put water in a clear bottle in the sunshine for two days was astonished at the burning quality of the water, a reaction which remained the same during following tests.

It was an interesting experience for me when, during a recent lecture for colour therapists, I noticed how they were on the same wavelength and how successfully they harmonised colours with their patients. It sometimes makes me shiver when I see the misuse and abuse of colour in advertisements. Colour therapy is a scientific method for the treatment of health and the mysticism that surrounds its practice is totally unnecessary and undeserved. It is a fact that colour is linked to all kinds of vibratory issues and therefore is a part of life that we cannot escape. Finally, never forget that colour is a gift of Nature. The laws of light were appreciated by ancient philosophers and physicians, and who are we to deny them, when we can see that sunlight, as if by magic, is capable of producing such a varied spectrum of colours.

It is vitally important to choose the correct colours for treatment. For inflammation of the eye, light treatment is used. For deafness we use yellow and sometimes red to stimulate the circulation, and blue to alleviate pain and inflammation. Every colour has an effect on the different parts of the body where problems may arise. I would say that Nature's greatest gift is light as this without a doubt means life, to be closely followed by colour which serves to improve our health, as well as brightening our existence. Colour is life, and life is colour, and this can be seen in food. Once food has lost its colour, it has also lost its efficacy. Let's not underestimate the tremendous value of colour and I am sure that patients who have been treated with colour therapy will wholeheartedly agree with me.

IRIDOLOGY

I have often been asked by puzzled patients what I can see when I practise iridology. The eyes provide us with the fine-tuned analysis of biochemistry and of emotional and circumstantial factors which are hard to determine using any other method. Iridology is the science of analysing the delicate structures of the iris of the eye. Under the magnification of a biomicroscope the iris reveals itself as a world of minute detail, a complete map that represents a communication system capable of handling an amazing quantity of information.

The iris is an extension of the brain prolifically endowed with hundreds of thousands of nerve endings, microscopic blood vessels, muscle and other tissues. Each iris is connected to every organ and tissue of the body by way of the brain and nervous system. The nerve fibres receive their impulses by way of their connection to the optic nerve, optic thalmus and spinal cord. They are formed embryologically from mesoderm and neuroectoderm tissues, and both the sympathetic and parasympathetic nervous systems are present in the iris. By way of nerve reflex responses Nature has provided us with a miniature television screen showing the most remote parts of the body, which normally cannot be seen by conventional diagnostic methods.

To a qualified practitioner the eye presents a picture of the entire anatomy of the body. In the early 1800s an 11-year-old boy called Ignatz von Peczely became engaged in a struggle with a captured owl. With fierce claws the bird tried to defend itself. In their struggle the boy accidentally broke the owl's leg. While the youth and the owl glared into each other's eyes, the boy observed a black stripe appearing in the owl's eye. This black stripe eventually changed to a tiny black spot, surrounded by white lines and shadings. When von Peczely grew up he became a physician, but he never forgot the incident with the owl. Working on the surgical ward of the hospital gave him the opportunity to observe the irises of patients after accidents or injuries. This was the beginning of iridology, nearly two centuries ago, and since then it has progressed and grown into a valuable science.

The iris of the eye is a most complex tissue, but by observation of the iris, one can detect many problems scientifically, some of which are deeply buried. There are areas of lightness that occur on the surface, set against discoloured areas, that will tell the practitioner what is going on. The constitution of the eye will reveal much about the state of the patient's health and the colour of the iris in all its variety will often remind the practitioner of the seven colours of the rainbow and disclose whether there is harmony or disharmony. I mostly look for specifics: for example, the eyes of a cancer patient usually show a very clear picture of the destruction that is being wreaked within the body. Every cell, organ and tissue has its history and iridology points out weaknesses and alerts the practitioner to their existence.

Dr Nico Bos was one of the first and foremost Dutch practitioners in the field of iridology. He taught me and he often told me that iris diagnosis is a form of diagnosis that requires love and interest on the part of the practitioner. Some claims that are made about iridology are not true, and unfortunately some so-called practitioners use it in an indiscriminate manner. What it does reveal is the strength and weaknesses in the patient's health and also any nutritional and chemical needs the patient may have. It reveals the body in its entirety as a unified structure, allowing practitioners to define catarrhal conditions, acid/alkaline situations, the nerve force, toxic accumulation and other more general health issues.

It should be remembered that iridology does not show specific diseases; it does, however, reveal scars. A female patient recently professed that she had no faith in iridology. When I examined her eyes and asked her what was wrong with her right kidney, she doubtfully responded by asking me if I was clairvoyant. When I denied this she querulously enquired how it was possible for me to know that she had lost her right kidney many years ago. I read this in her eyes, and the lady admitted that she had to reconsider her long-held belief that iridology was a sinecure.

Iridology, or the science of iris diagnosis, will pinpoint exactly where the lymphatics are deranged in a patient, and which organ or organs. This obviates any guesswork and searching over the body. Study of the lymphatic chain in the iris will assist a competent practitioner in his or her diagnosis, and as the compass is to the captain of a ship, so iridology will prove to be invaluable in locating the blocked sea of lymph and its channels.

The collectively named lymphatic nodes include the following:

- Cervical lymph nodes
- Auxilliary lymph nodes
- Mammary lymph nodes
- Thoracic lymph nodes
- Abdominal lymph nodes (3 branches)
- Inguinal lymph nodes
- Popliteal lymph nodes

OTHER TREATMENT METHODS
Light, colour and iridology are all very helpful therapies in the

treatment of vision. However, there are other treatment methods that may be applied to vision problems, one of which is laser treatment. This is also a form of light, and with this method it is possible to restore tissue, and when the laser is used on acupuncture points, it can be of great benefit. Furthermore, acupuncture treatment can also be applied, depending on the nature of the condition. Osteopathy, and especially cranial osteopathy, is very influential on the endocrine system, and this is therefore an equally useful tool.

How do we safeguard our vision? In common with general health care I must stipulate that diet, exercise and plenty of fresh air are essential. Having read this chapter, however, you will know that in the specific case of vision problems, there are a number of therapies and treatment methods that can be applied and that one must never give up hope.

CASE HISTORIES

Remaining true to the format of this book, I will now continue with some case histories. An elderly gentleman had nearly lost his sight. He was a pianist and found that now he was only able to play from memory, because he could no longer read his music. I decided on acupuncture combined with laser treatment. I also prescribed the Bioforce remedy Euphrasiasan, which is a combination remedy based on eyebright and specifically designed for the treatment of conjunctivitis and general eye problems. It has also been used successfully in the treatment of blepharitis, which is inflammation of the edges of the eyelids including the hair follicles and glands. The recommended dose is five drops in a glass of water, to be drunk at odd intervals during the day, a few sips at a time. The versatility of this remedy is such that it may also be used externally: a few drops can be placed on the closed eyelid and massaged in gently until absorbed and the fluid has dried.

Because this patient's calcium levels were low I prescribed Urticalcin from Bioforce, which is an easily absorbable calcium (five tablets, twice daily). I supplemented this with *Calc. fluor* x3 (two tablets, twice daily). My patient reacted to the treatment with surprising speed and his sight was largely restored. He was brimming over with gratitude and happiness when he found he was able to read music again.

Then there was a young female patient, in her mid-twenties, with blepharitis. One did not need to be a diagnostical genius to recognise the problem. The inflammation of the eyelids was only too clear: they were red and thickened, with the formation of scales, crusts and small ulcers. Ulcerated blepharitis is usually caused by a bacterial infection and can be quite difficult to overcome. However, she responded excellently when I prescribed a high dosage of Echinaforce (twenty-five drops in some water, twice daily), together with fifteen drops of Emergency Essence twice daily and the Bioforce herbal remedy *Galeopsis*, and finally a strong vitamin C supplement. She was full of appreciation, because her self-confidence had been given a severe knock by the reactions of people who did not know her, as her problems had been very visible to all.

A gentleman aged thirty-four presented me with an acute conjunctivitis. This is an inflammation brought on by a virus, bacteria or an allergy. In this case I suspected that it was a side-effect of hay fever. I used Pollinosan, which was specifically designed by Dr Vogel for the treatment of hay fever, and I also prescribed an Enzymatic Therapy remedy called I-Tone. This remedy recognises the importance of vitamin A in eye function. It also contains many other important nutrients, including vitamin C, which plays a critical role in capillary development. Capillaries are tiny blood vessels that carry oxygen and nutrients to cells, and the eyes are rich in capillaries. Antioxidant nutrients such as betacarotene protect the eyes and other organs against free radicals. The body uses B vitamins (such as niacin, riboflavin and inositol) in nervous system functions. More nerve cells are devoted to eyesight than to any other sense. I-Tone combines these nutrients with herbal extracts of alfalfa, eyebright and greater celandine. To complete the treatment I prescribed a Swiss eyedrop called Occulosan, which is an extremely effective remedy for cleansing the eyes.

I was presented with an unusual, but interesting case by a long-distance lorry driver, aged forty-four, whose sight was slowly but certainly diminishing. When I examined and questioned him I came to my conclusion when I learned that he was a fervent pipe smoker, and in the habit of allowing the pipe to dangle from the right corner of his mouth. I was able to deduce this because his right eye was very much worse than his left eye and I had witnessed before the general degeneration of sight with heavy smokers. This patient's sight was greatly improved when he started to use the remedy Vision Essentials. This remedy is largely based on bilberry. The use of bilberry has been found to be highly effective in cases of diabetic retinopathy, macular degeneration, cataracts and glaucoma. Bilberry, perhaps better known in Europe as the blueberry – *Vaccinium myrtillus* – is a member of the *Vaccinium* family that comprises nearly 200 species of berries (including the cranberry). Bilberry has great medical properties and the pharmacologically active constituents are flavonoid compounds known as anthocyanocites. Bilberries not only have great nutritional value, but some of their medicinal properties make them an effective remedy for scurvy and urinary complaints.

It was remarkable how well my patient recovered with the treatment prescribed. In other instances I have seen how effective Vision Essentials can be in the treatment of retinitis pigmentosa and also for night-blindness.

An elderly lady suffered eye injuries during a road accident. To strengthen the eyes a vitamin supplement is always advisable and I prescribed Health Insurance Plus (one tablet, twice daily), Emergency Essence (fifteen drops, twice daily) and, as her circulation left something to be desired, she also took *Gingko biloba* (fifteen drops, twice a day). The side-effects of the injury were soon a thing of the past.

The next history was an extreme case. A 28-year-old man unfortunately suffered from macular degeneration. The macula is the portion of the eye responsible for fine vision. Degeneration of the macula is the leading cause of visual loss in persons aged fifty-five years and older. He was quite upset when I first saw him as his eyes were in quite a bad state and he was aware of the degeneration. His wife was expecting their first baby and he had been advised to undergo surgery, which he could not contemplate because of his religious beliefs.

From the outset we agreed that he should not have any false hopes. We embarked upon acupuncture and cranial osteopathy treatment sessions, as well as light and colour therapy. I also prescribed some remedies: *Petasites*, which is an extract of the plant butterbur, Urticalcin, *Galeopsis* and *Silicia* x3. I also prescribed beta carotene, vitamin C and Selenium from Nature's Best. He slowly but gradually improved. Somehow, the press heard of the story and a Manchester newspaper featured his story, with a photograph of my patient being able to see and holding his newborn daughter. He was a very happy man and believed that he had really experienced a miracle. I reassured him that the remedies, combined with his determination, had resulted in his regained sight. Macular degeneration is a hard condition to treat and it was impossible to predict with any certainty such a fortunate outcome.

One of the ladies on my staff who helped out when we were shorthanded suffered from glaucoma and complained of considerable discomfort. The glaucoma was of a chronic nature and there was little or no reaction to the orthodox treatment she was receiving from her GP. She was already on a high daily intake of vitamin C (2 g per day), and I also prescribed Vision Essentials and Arterioforce capsules, which reduced the pressure. She still uses the remedies and is convinced that these are largely responsible for a great reduction in the discomfort she had been experiencing. She is also inclined to believe that her eyesight has improved, and this gives us hope that she will be able to continue to control her problem.

I examined a 21-year-old girl and diagnosed retinitis pigmentosa, a condition of a slowly progressive bilateral retinal degeneration. Quite often this is hereditary and there is no known cure for this condition. However, I knew that in some cases enzyme therapy has been beneficial and this I prescribed, combined with Vision Essentials. Unfortunately, the girl was also diabetic and because she was insulin-dependent I advised her to take a chromium supplement from Lamberts Healthcare called Chromium 200 (one capsule daily). The manufacturer's recommendation is that Chromium 200 may play a part in enabling the cells to take up glucose for energy release and for the synthesis of fatty acids and cholesterol.

A male patient in his late twenties had a corneal ulcer. His hobby was clay pigeon-shooting and his eye condition was obviously of great concern to him. He had been informed that there was not much to be done and I could not give him much hope either. However, with laser and acupuncture treatment, together with Emergency Essence and bilberry extract, he fortunately improved. Recently, I saw him and he proudly showed me an impressive list of his scores at clay pigeon-shooting.

A female patient in her mid-seventies who had a cataract called on me for help. There are two kinds of cataract, green and grey, and both are fairly common. I advised that she take *Gingko biloba* because of its great results with circulation problems and Vitality Essence from the flower remedies. Vision Essentials, with its bilberry ingredient, was also very helpful. Fortunately, the remedies were effective in this lady's case, and although she is not totally cured, she has improved a great deal.

In the *American Journal of Natural Medicine* I read that cataracts are the leading cause of impaired vision and blindness in the United States. Approximately four million people have some degree of vision-impairing cataract, and at least 40,000 people in the United States are blind due to cataracts. Cataracts are a source of tremendous financial burden on our society and cataract surgery is the most common surgical procedure done in the United States each year (600,000 per annum) for patients on Medicare at a cost of over $4 billion.

Bilberry anthocyanosides may offer significant protection against the development of cataracts. The occurrence of cataracts in rats can be reduced by changing their diet from a commercial laboratory feed to a 'well-defined diet'. Preliminary research suggests that flavonoid components in the well-defined diets may be responsible for the protective effects.

In one human study, bilberry extract plus vitamin E stopped the progression of cataract formation in 97 per cent of a group of fifty patients with senile cortical cataracts.

Depending on the patient's condition, some of the remedies

mentioned in this chapter have resulted in new hope, even for some of those who had been told that there was not much reason left for hope, and yet they refused to give up. We must understand that it is Nature that is the healer, and not man. Nature provides man with the means of seeking a solution to their problem, if only we know where to look. In fact, we do no more than try to support the body's ability for natural self-healing. This is the basic principle of natural remedies and we can only be grateful that we are instrumental in this process.

Conclusion

During late 1996 and early 1997 I have lost a lot of dear friends. Two of them were also my best teachers, Dr Alfred Vogel and Dr Leonard Allan. Both of them, in their lifetime, preached the gospel of health and have shown many ways in which we can help and protect ourselves. Dr Allan left me his entire library, which contains a wealth of knowledge, a gift for which I am extremely grateful. I have not been able to work through all of his books left to me, but already in some of those I have had time to study, I have read about the warning signs which are so obvious in today's society. Good health is a real challenge for all of us.

I worked with Dr Alfred Vogel for almost forty years and his most valuable present was the gift of himself: his friendship, his life and knowledge. I visited him not long before he died and during one of our last conversations he still showed concern about the world's ignorance about obstacles to health. He still passionately cared about telling people how they could help themselves to good health. When it was time for me to return to Britain, he embraced me and we said our goodbyes. Before I left he presented me with his final gift: a set of big books which he had used nearly all his life. These books were written by Dr Manfred Curry during the 1930s and Dr Vogel invariably referred to these books when he needed guidance on the treatment of patients.

These books are packed with advice on how to keep ourselves healthy, and they also mention the five senses and how they are influenced by atmosphere and pollution. Every day we meet people who have problems with touch, loss of eyesight, impaired hearing, or have lost either their sense of smell or taste. Many of these problems are the result of what was forecast in these books. Because these books are written in German I have to read slowly, but I want to understand the message that is contained in them. It is a message I want to share with others.

Five of those friends that I have lost in the past three months were also respected colleagues. They all left more than earthly possessions or books. They all left behind examples of hard work, understanding and a love of helping others, either physically, mentally or spiritually. I felt the loss of each of them sharply, including that of one of my organic gardeners, who understood Nature as well as any of my learned friends. With their examples in mind, I feel an even greater challenge to do better and to help others.

There is an extra sense, which is so mysteriously talked about, and about which most people have their own opinion. Yet who is to say what it was that alerted the pilot during the landing that could have been fateful, and how does the migrating bird instinctively know where it should be heading?

Years ago I read a German book written by Dietrich Gumbel, who made some very interesting observations regarding the senses. He too understood the message of herbal medicine, flower essences, their characteristics and their signature. He even explained holistically how the three layers of the skin reflect the three-dimensional appearance of a human being, and he calls skin the 'sense of life'. He stated in his book that all sense organs, which are conscious organs, are developed in a way that imparts consciousness, which is a condition of the mind to the human being. Mind and consciousness are inseparable and merely two sides of the same coin.

The development and significance of the sense organs have a double origin because these organs are built as a mutually organised penetration of nervous tissue, with messages from the brain and the epidermis. Both of these tissues, however, have the same parent tissue, which is derived from the ectoderm. These five organs have an awareness and a consciousness in the function of the sense organs: the ear is a mental sense organ; smelling through the nose is stimulating the respiratory system; seeing is the comprehension of light, and the eyes take in light energy; the ears respond to electromagnetic frequencies; and food intake takes place through the mouth.

During the third week of embryonic development there is a primary ectodermal buccal fossa upwardly folded into a pouch, the so-called Ratke Pouch. This is developed in a glandular sac with a short exit to the buccal cavity and intermingles with the primordium at the skull base. This hypophyseal duct is stressed into a canal which later disappears. The remainder exists as a small glandular hypophysis pharyngae on the superior wall of the pharynx on the external wall of the sphenoid bone, a function which is still unknown. The skin plays a tremendous role in this and the sensory organs and is developed as an innovation of three nerve endings. The eye, the eardrum, the nose and the mouth are developed in this way.

The hypophysis cerebri is another name for the pituitary gland, and is said to be responsible for the sixth sense in man. What is the reason for this sixth sense? It is interesting to note that in some twentieth-century diseases, such as ME, the hypophysis and inner sensory organs do not seem able to maintain or control levels of hormones in the bloodstream. The sixth sense is often referred to with an air of mystery. In the animal kingdom it is known as instinct and in the human world the equivalent is intuition. It is worth remembering that in some people intuition is more highly developed than in others. Dr Dietrich Gumbel wrote that the hypophysis cerebri or pituitary gland is the centre for consciousness and self-awareness in the human being.

Man has not one but three bodies, and these three bodies have to be in harmony for the senses to function properly. When you lose one of these senses you lose your sense of living. The *New Scientist* recently featured an article called 'The Sixth Sense' and the commercial world is trying to exploit this idea. The five tangible senses are easy to explain. The article suggests that the sixth sense is no more than a sex organ. Researchers remain sceptical about the prospect. Other scientists believe it exists and it has been recorded that many years ago alchemists tried to manufacture a special scent that attracted women, not only for use as a perfume, but also to treat pre-menstrual tension. The article states that men will be attracted when the sense of smell is stimulated by the female pheromone and before long they will be able to manufacture the pheromone for the commercial market. For centuries man has only been able to guess the truth. Will we ever discover the truth or are the secrets of Nature still locked into the secrets of Creation? It is quite obvious that there are more things in heaven and earth than are dreamt of in our philosophy, as William Shakespeare wrote in *Hamlet*. Is our holistic system of mind, body and spirit, open to discover the secrets of Creation and are we ready for any discovery? Would it not be wiser to look around and see what we can discover on our own planet instead of shooting rockets to explore the moon? Think of the powers of the caperberry which are now harnessed in Vitality Essence, and provide extra energy and vitality. Keep in mind *Hypericum perforatum*, or St John's wort, the main constituent of Hyperiforce, which is so widely used and relied upon. Surely these remedies deserve a place in a world where only too often people are in danger of losing touch with reality.

I felt very sorry when I realised how confused a female patient was and I decided to take a Kirlian photograph of her hands. The result was intriguing and the photograph displayed two electromagnetic auras – this was something I had never seen before. We spoke for quite some time and I learned that she believed herself to be possessed. A remedy based on the fresh extract of *Hypericum perforatum* combined with a great deal of discussions helped this lady to refind her mental balance.

Creation is holistic and man must live in harmony with the plant world as well as the animal kingdom, so that one day we will live in peace and unity, enabling us to enjoy freedom.

The other day I saw a patient who complained of a constant burning sensation in the mouth, having lost his senses of smell and taste, while his vision had also become impaired. With the help of some herbal remedies he cured himself. Sometimes the answers really are simple, if we only know where to look. He wisely focused on happiness when he practised relaxation exercises. Visualisation can help us to regain our individuality and focus on the more important things in life. Every day I try to follow the principles of prayer and meditation to discover the right direction.

Some time ago I attended a large exhibition in Germany on all kinds of aspects of medicine, where I came across large numbers of new remedies and medicines. My eye was drawn to a very simple stand, perhaps even the smallest of the entire exhibition, where I saw a display of Propolis preparations. Propolis is produced by bees; it is a substance that contains strong antioxidants, antibacterials and flavonoids. Bees produce this mixture from the pollen of trees and flowers and use it to seal and build their hives. Patients with viral activity have greatly benefited from the use of Propolis K and Bee Propolis. Propolis K should be taken on a piece of bread (about ten drops) which should be chewed thoroughly. This will disinfect the mucous membranes, the throat and saliva.

There is so much talk today about viruses, parasites and bacteria, that we would do well to remember that they have been in existence an awful lot longer than we have and are constantly increasing in strength, while our immune system is becoming weaker. Life is a constant warfare between healthy and diseased cells. The stronger we make the healthy cell, the more we are likely to overcome the sick or diseased cells.

Through following the guidance we are offered, and keeping an open mind, we find many ways to help other people. Occasionally I have been nicknamed 'the man with the X-ray eyes'. This is not because I might be endowed with ultra-perceptive capabilities, but because I try and keep my vision clear and allow myself to be led by the divine spirit of our Creator, who will always help if we ask. Maintaining a strong belief allows us a security which is beyond explanation. I thank God every morning when I awake for the tremendous gift of being able to help others. Life, tradition and history is changing fast, but we have the security of knowing that we are protected by that great love which is within us all. It is manifested in more ways than we can see with the human eye. Light is the medicine of the future, but we can only use it if we are in harmony with cosmic light.

Whilst on this subject, I am immediately reminded of some patients who had lost not only the powers of speech, touch and taste, but also muscle strength, and it was clear in their case that life was ebbing away. When one particular patient, however, showed some unexpected improvement, I learned about a treatment he had received from a New Zealand doctor. Dr Brooker, a medical as well as naturopathic doctor, was a genius who had studied light, colour and magnetic fields. This patient, who suffered from motor neurone disease, had lost the power of speech, but noticed a gradual return after having visited Dr Brooker for treatment. When I investigated further I learned that Dr Brooker treated his patients with electric currents. He would vary the points of contact on the body, depending on the problems concerned. It all seemed to be too simple to be true, but I realised immediately what Dr Brooker was doing: by touching important energy points on the body, causing a vibration, he was breaking down blockages in the flow of energy. We are fortunate that Dr Brooker shared his knowledge, but he died before completing this task. A small group of British scientists have studied his methods in greater detail and have been conducting trials at a London hospital. These trials into the effects of a vibratory pulse on viruses and energy blockages are now about to be concluded and it is hoped that from their findings we will learn more about restoring harmony in the body energy.

Dr George W. Crile was a surgeon during the First World War. At that time he observed that death often resulted from shell shock or other forms of trauma, despite the fact that there was no ascertainable structural damage to vital organs. His first major conclusions appeared in his book *A Bi-Polar Theory of Living Processes*. He was convinced that life is a bi-polar electrical phenomenon and suggested that in the human body the brain is the positive pole, and the liver the negative pole. He observed that in an embryo the brain and liver are the first organs to be differentiated. Destroy one, and the other dies. His evidence for the negative polarity of the liver was that it collects metallic poisons, as metals are electrically positive.

Later, he expanded the concept of the negative pole to include the voluntary muscles and red blood cells as well as the lining of the blood vessel walls. He maintained that red blood cells are constantly generating negative electricity by virtue of friction against the walls of the vessels. Parasympathetic pathways convey negative charges to the brain.

On the cellular level he noted that the nucleus and cytoplasm are the positive and negative poles respectively. The germ cells are special cases: the ovum is largely cytoplasm, while the sperm cell is mainly nucleus. The impregnated ovum represents a potential difference well in excess of that to be found in an ordinary tissue cell. Dr Crile believed that his double energy accounted for the rapid cell multiplication manifested in embryonic development. This theory is applicable even to the bacterial cell, which has no visible nucleus. He reasoned that such a cell is actually all nucleus, but its negative pole is provided by the alkaline environment in which it lives. This explains why bacteria are likely to be destroyed by acids.

What have we learned about nerves? It has been established that nerves are surrounded by electromagnetic fields. Plexus areas are markedly positive. If a nerve is cut, but not otherwise damaged, a weak, but measurable, electric current flows along the fibre in both directions from the point of severance. It is a smooth flow, not the pulsating flow of the nerve impulse. By tampering with a nerve fibre it is possible to modify the electrical characteristics of the nerve cell wall. It is part of a data transmission network.

The effects of magnetic fields on living organisms are many and varied. Flat worms, when confronted by a bar magnet, change direction. Polarity is reversed in sleep, coma, hypnosis and anaesthesia. Fields and currents are reversed by amputation and surgery. The earth's energy interacts with energy in the body to create equilibrium between the body and its biomagnetic activity. This results in the restoration of health. Most disease is the result of *excess* energy, as opposed to insufficient energy.

Magnetic fields have always existed. Restoring and harmonising energy through magnetic fields is practised in many different ways. Even the touch of a thumb can play an important part in restoring energy and harmony. What is illness? Or, for that matter, what is health? Without doubt, illness is disharmony, and health is dynamic equilibrium, when the three bodies of man – physical, mental and emotional – are in balance. From training in acupuncture we know that given points can be influenced positively by touch, and in some instances by injection or acupuncture needles.

Neural therapy, developed by Professor Huneke, has shown that by injecting an acupuncture point with a natural substance, pain can be relieved, often more effectively than by using cortisone injections. There is a right time, place and point for everything.

The Papyrus of Ebers was written in 1552 BC and this is the first known record of medicine. Before that time tinctures and oils were used medicinally, and from this document we learn that there were about seven hundred remedies at the time of writing, but they were often difficult to apply or take. Ancient records also exist that reveal advanced medical knowledge for that era compiled by a Greek pharmacist named Galenus von Pergamon, who lived in Rome during the second century after Christ. Centuries passed until the Arabian Doctor Rhazes (AD 865–925) discovered a pill. Problems arose as the pill was insoluble in the bowels, and history repeated itself with the Persian Ayicanna (AD 980–1037) who formulated pills using gold and silver, which were found to be equally useless. During the nineteenth century advanced innovations included a soft gelatin capsule developed by Mothes of France in 1834, while in 1843 an Englishman, Brickdon, patented a tablet which greatly improved matters. Since then there has been an explosion in the numbers of new drugs available. Countless tests have been carried out in the name of science, in our never-ceasing attempts to improve medicine, though all too often they overlook the obvious.

The answer is simple. Look at the fresh herbs, flowers and plants that surround us, even roots and the bark on the trees. Appreciate their individual characteristics and know that these may be employed for the good of mankind. Fresh beetroot is a naturally effective antioxidant; a raw potato filters bodily acid and a cabbage leaf compress on an arthritic joint will bring relief. Simple remedies they may be, but they are effective. Please do not disregard them as old wives' tales. These remedies are gifts from Nature and who are we to ignore them as being insufficiently sophisticated? Let me stress that anything supplied by Nature should be used in its freshest possible state, and bear in mind that holistic and natural treatments complement each other.

Honour must be given to all physicians and scientists who have had such influence on the development of medicine, but above all to our Creator, who always fulfilled His promise of food to enable us to exist and herbs for healing. It would sometimes appear as if mankind is intent on destroying himself and the planet. We must decide if we feel that we belong to Nature, or if science has caused us to lose our ability to think biologically. Today's lifespan has increased enormously, largely because of scientific developments, but let us not overlook the importance of the quality of life. What we see is a rather depressing picture of a radical increase in progressive, degenerative disease. The ideal solution would be for orthodox scientific methods to work with the old trusted methods, and we would have a better system. It is high time that these two facets of medicine worked together to overcome the problems that we face today. An old Spanish saying that if you want to grow old you must start young, contains a great deal of common sense. Prevention is better than cure, and it is only by following a sensible diet, controlling stress, taking regular exercise and maintaining a well-balanced blood pressure, that we have a chance to protect ourselves.

Many years ago, after my graduation as a pharmacist, I was invited for an interview at a major pharmaceutical manufacturer in the Netherlands. When I toured the factory, I was not only impressed to see all the drugs that were produced there, I was appalled. Little do we think about the destruction of animals for the sake of the manufacture of drugs. That day I questioned whether I really wanted to be part of that. I fully accept that some of the medicines manufactured in this way are most definitely essential to save lives. How fortunate I was, however, to meet Dr Alfred Vogel, who influenced my perception of natural medicine, showed me new possibilities and changed my life. I asked for clear vision, and I am sure it was my meeting with Dr Vogel that opened my eyes to what Nature has to offer us.

Neither technology, medicine nor hygiene can stop the advances of time. As we get older it is inevitable that we will experience more problems with our health, and therefore we must look for ways to protect the quality of our life. The five tangible senses will serve as a reminder that none of us are as young as we once were. Is it indeed true that the advancement of technology and science has extracted too high a price in that pollution has impaired our senses of touch, taste, vision, smell and hearing? Think seriously about this and decide whether the time has now come to sound the alarm because, if we lose our senses, we lose our sense of living!

Bibliography

Ackerman, Diane. *The Natural History of the Senses*, Phoenix, London
Bartram, Thomas. *Encyclopedia of Herbal Medicine*, Grace Publishing, Christchurch, Dorset
Benjamin, Harry. *Everybody's Guide – The Natural Cure*, Thorsons Publishing, Wellingborough, Northants
Clark, Linda. *Colon Therapy*, The Devin Adair Co., Connecticut
Cowan, David and Girdlestone, Rodney. *Safe as Houses*, Gateway Books, Bath, UK
Curry, Dr Manfred. *Bioklimatik*, American Bioclimatic Research Institute, Rieder, Ammersee, Germany
Davis, Andrew P. *Neuropathy*, Graves and Hessey, Long Beach, California
Gazella, Karolyn A. *Help Yourself*, Impact Comm. Inc.
Gimbel, Theo. *The Colour Therapy*, Element, Shaftesbury, Dorset
Guradas. *Flower Essences*, Brotherhood of Life, Albuquerque, New Mexico
Hanish, Dr O.Z.A. *The Power of Health*, Mazdaznan Press, Los Angeles, USA
Kroeger, Hanna. *God Helps Those That Help Themselves*, Hanna Kroeger
Lieberman, Jacob. *Light – Medicine of the Future*, Bear & Co., Santa Fe, New Mexico
Mansfield, Peter. *The Bates Method*, Vermillion, London
Martin, Gill. *Aromatherapy*, McDonald & Co., London
Serrentino, Jo. *Natural Remedies Work*, Hartley and Marks, Washington, USA
Tappon, Francis M. *Massage Techniques*, The MacMillan Company, New York
Vogel, Dr A. *The Nature Doctor*, Mainstream Publishing, Edinburgh
White, Ian. *Bush Flower Essences*, Bantam Books, Sydney, New York, London
Woodhouse, E.E. *One Man's Dictionary of Sense*, Swift Limited, Albion Place, London EC1

Useful Addresses

Auchenkyle, Southwoods Road, Troon, Ayrshire KA10 7EL
Bach Flower Remedies, Unit 6, Suffolk Way, Abingdon, Oxon OX14 5JX
Bioforce UK Ltd, Olympic Business Park, Dundonald, Ayrshire KA2 9BE
Bioforce Canada Ltd, 11 German Street, Newmarket, Ontario L3Y 7V1
Bioforce USA Ltd, Kinderhook, New York, USA
Britannia Health Products Ltd, Forum House, Brighton Road, Redhill, Surrey RH1 6YS
British Acupuncture Association, 34 Alderney Street, London SW1V 4EU
Enzymatic Therapy, Hadley Wood Healthcare, 67a Beech Hill, Hadley Wood, Barnet, Herts EN4 0JW
Enzymatic Therapy, PO Box 22310, Green Bay W1 54305, USA
General Council and Register of Naturopaths, Frazer House, 6 Netherhall Gardens, London NW3 5RR
General Council and Register of Osteopaths, 56 London Street, Reading, Berks RG1 4SQ
Hadley Wood Healthcare, 67a Beech Hill, Hadley Wood, Barnet, Herts EN4 0JW
Montana, Hadley Wood Healthcare, 67a Beech Hill, Hadley Wood, Barnet, Herts EN4 0JW
Nature's Best, Dept. HT01, 1 Lamberts Road, Tunbridge Wells, Kent TH2 3EQ
A. Nelson & Co. Ltd, 5 Endeavour Way, Wimbledon, London SW19 9UH
Obbekjaers, 209 Blackburn Road, Wheelton, Chorley, Lancs
Sans Souci, Hadley Wood Healthcare, 67a Beech Hill, Hadley Wood, Barnet, Herts EN4 0JW